SleepWell:
Pediatrics, Psychiatry and Neurology

Vol. 3

SleepWell:

Pediatrics, Psychiatry and Neurology

Vol. 3

Edited by:

Janice D. Key, MD
Associate Professor of Pediatrics
Director of Adolescent Medicine
Medical University of South Carolina
Charleston, South Carolina

D. Walter Hiott, MD
Assistant Professor of Psychiatry
Medical University of South Carolina
Attending Psychiatrist
Ralph H. Johnson VA Medical Center
Charleston, South Carolina

Timothy D. Carter, MD
Associate Professor of Neurology
Neurology Residency Program Director
Clinical Neurophysiology Fellowship Director
Medical University of South Carolina
Charleston, South Carolina

Series Editors:

Benjamin Clyburn, MD
Assistant Professor of Medicine
Internal Medicine Residency Program Director
Medical University of South Carolina
Charleston, South Carolina

George J. Taylor, MD
Professor of Medicine
Medical University of South Carolina
Charleston, South Carolina

Blackwell
Publishing

© 2003 by Blackwell Science
a Blackwell Publishing company

Blackwell Publishing, Inc., 350 Main Street, Malden, Massachusetts 02148-5018, USA
Blackwell Science Ltd, Osney Mead, Oxford OX2 0EL, UK
Blackwell Science Asia Pty Ltd, 550 Swanston Street, Carlton South, Victoria 3053, Australia
Blackwell Verlag GmbH, Kurfürstendamm 57, 10707 Berlin, Germany

All rights reserved. No part of this publication may be reproduced in any form or by any electronic or mechanical means, including information storage and retrieval systems, without permission in writing from the publisher, except by a reviewer who may quote brief passages in a review.

02 03 04 05   5 4 3 2 1

ISBN: 0-632-04666-X

Library of Congress Cataloging-in-Publication Data

Sleepwell. Volume 3, Pediatrics, psychiatry, and neurology / edited by Janice D. Key, D. Walter Hiott, Timothy D. Carter.
   p. ; cm.
   ISBN 0-632-04666-X (pbk.)
   1. Neurology—Examinations, questions, etc.   2. Psychiatry—Examinations, questions, etc.   3. Pediatrics—Examinations, questions, etc.
   4. Physicians—Licenses—United States—Examinations—Study guides.   I. Key, Janice D.   II. Hiott, D. Walter.   III. Carter, Timothy D.
   IV. Title: Pediatrics, psychiatry, and neurology.
   [DNLM: 1. Pediatrics—Examination Questions.   2. Mental Disorders—Examination Questions.
3. Nervous System Diseases—Examination Questions.   WS 18.2 S6323 2002]
   RC343.5.S544 2002
   616.8–dc21

2002009536

A catalogue record for this title is available from the British Library

Acquisitions: Beverly Copland
Development: Angela Gagliano
Production: Debra Lally
Cover design: Leslie Haimes
Interior design: Mary McKeon
Typesetter: TechBooks in York, PA
Printed and bound by Sheridan Books in Ann Arbor, MI

For further information on Blackwell Publishing, visit our website:
www.medirect.com

Notice: The indications and dosages of all drugs in this book have been recommended in the medical literature and conform to the practices of the general community. The medications described and treatment prescriptions suggested do not necessarily have specific approval by the Food and Drug Administration for use in the diseases and dosages for which they are recommended. The package insert for each drug should be consulted for use and dosage as approved by the FDA. Because standards for usage change, it is advisable to keep abreast of revised recommendations, particularly those concerning new drugs.

Contents

SECTION 1: PEDIATRICS • 1

Case 1: **Infant with tachypnea**—*Douglas E. Halbert, MD* • 2
Case 2: **Toddler with cough**—*Douglas E. Halbert, MD* • 3
Case 3: **Toddler with recurrent cough**—*Douglas E. Halbert, MD* • 4
Case 4: **Preschool child with a rash**—*Douglas E. Halbert, MD* • 5
Case 5: **Preschool child with a seizure**—*Douglas E. Halbert, MD* • 6
Case 6: **Adolescent with weakness**—*Douglas E. Halbert, MD* • 7
Case 7: **Adolescent with pneumonia**—*Douglas E. Halbert, MD* • 8
Case 8: **Toddler with ear pain**—*Douglas E. Halbert, MD* • 9
Case 9: **Adolescent with headache and papilledema**—*Douglas E. Halbert, MD* • 10
Case 10: **Preschool child with weight loss and lymphadenopathy**—*Douglas E. Halbert, MD* • 11
Case 11: **Toddler with developmental delay**—*Tina B. Stewart, MD* • 12
Case 12: **Thrombocytopenia**—*Douglas E. Halbert, MD* • 13
Case 13: **Adolescent with vaginal bleeding**—*Janice D. Key, MD* • 14
Case 14: **School-age child with an abnormal gait**—*Douglas E. Halbert, MD* • 15
Case 15: **Illness in a neonate**—*Tina B. Stewart, MD* • 16
Case 16: **Cough and headache**—*Douglas E. Halbert, MD* • 17
Case 17: **School failure in an adolescent**—*Janice D. Key* • 18
Case 18: **Scrotal pain in a prepubertal boy**—*Tina B. Stewart, MD* • 20
Case 19: **Infant with a murmur**—*Douglas E. Halbert, MD* • 21
Case 20: **Infant with wheezing**—*Douglas E. Halbert, MD* • 22
Case 21: **Urinary tract infection**—*Tina B. Stewart, MD* • 23
Case 22: **Varicella (chicken pox)**—*Tina B. Stewart, MD* • 24
Case 23: **Enlarged tonsils and adenoids**—*Janice D. Key, MD* • 25
Case 24: **Ingestion**—*Tina B. Stewart, MD* • 26
Case 25: **School failure in a 9-year-old**—*Janice D. Key, MD* • 27
Case 26: **Rhinorrhea**—*Tina B. Stewart, MD* • 28
Case 27: **Anemia in a toddler**—*Janice D. Key, MD* • 29
Case 28: **Adolescent with weight loss**—*Janice D. Key, MD* • 30
Case 29: **Asthma**—*Tina B. Stewart, MD* • 31
Case 30: **Short Stature**—*Tina B. Stewart, MD* • 33
Case 31: **Fatigue in an adolescent**—*Janice D. Key, MD* • 36
Case 32: **Infant with developmental delay**—*Tina B. Stewart, MD* • 38
Case 33: **Infant with dysmorphic features**—*Janice D. Key, MD* • 39

Case 34: Recurrent wheezing and pneumonia—*Janice D. Key, MD* • **40**
Case 35: Poor growth in a toddler—*Janice D. Key, MD* • **41**
Case 36: Diarrhea in a toddler—*Janice D. Key, MD* • **44**
Case 37: Immunizations in childhood—*Janice D. Key, MD* • **45**
Case 38: Fever and rash in a preschool child—*Janice D. Key, MD* • **46**
Case 39: Primary amenorrhea—*Janice D. Key, MD* • **47**
Case 40: Knee pain in an adolescent boy—*Janice D. Key, MD* • **48**
Case 41: Growth and development in an adolescent—*Janice D. Key, MD* • **49**
Case 42: Respiratory distress in a neonate—*Janice D. Key, MD* • **50**
Case 43: Strabismus in a toddler—*Janice D. Key, MD* • **51**
Case 44: Dehydration in a child—*Valerie M. Panzarino, MD* • **52**
Case 45: Abdominal pain and bloody diarrhea—*Valerie M. Panzarino, MD* • **53**
Case 46: A child with swelling—*Valerie M. Panzarino, MD* • **54**
Case 47: Crush injury in a child—*Valerie M. Panzarino, MD* • **55**
Case 48: Joint pain in an adolescent—*Valerie M. Panzarino, MD* • **56**
Case 49: Toddler with stridor—*Douglas E. Halbert, MD* • **57**
Case 50: Infant with fever—*Douglas E. Halbert, MD* • **58**

SECTION 2: PSYCHIATRY • 59

Case 51: Behavioral disturbance of childhood—*Mary C. Fields, MD* • **60**
Case 52: Attention deficit/hyperactivity disorder—*Mary C. Fields, MD* • **61**
Case 53: Eating disorders—*Mary C. Fields, MD* • **62**
Case 54: Child sexual abuse—*Michael A. de Arellano, PhD & D. Walter Hiott, MD* • **63**
Case 55: Developmental, gender, and cultural considerations in major depressive disorder in children—*Michael A. de Arellano, PhD & D. Walter Hiott, MD* • **64**
Case 56: Consequences of a sexual assault—*Michael A. de Arellano, PhD & D. Walter Hiott, MD* • **65**
Case 57: Why can't little Johnny pay attention?—*Matthew S. Koval, MD* • **66**
Case 58: Bipolar patient comes to town—*Matthew S. Koval, MD* • **67**
Case 59: The reluctant schizophrenic—*Matthew S. Koval, MD* • **68**
Case 60: Improved symptoms but diminished quality of life—*Matthew S. Koval, MD* • **69**
Case 61: Youth patient with hemiplegia—*Himanshu P. Upadhyaya, MBBS, MS* • **70**
Case 62: Shortness of breath—*Himanshu P. Upadhyaya, MBBS, MS* • **71**
Case 63: Chronic back pain in primary care—*Himanshu P. Upadhyaya, MBBS, MS* • **72**
Case 64: Anxious check writer—*Jessica A. Whiteley, PhD & D. Walter Hiott, MD* • **73**
Case 65: Dog attack—*Jessica A. Whiteley, PhD & D. Walter Hiott, MD* • **74**
Case 66: Hand washer—*Jessica A. Whiteley, PhD & D. Walter Hiott, MD* • **75**
Case 67: Smoking and pregnancy—*Patricia L. Fiero, PhD & D. Walter Hiott, MD* • **76**
Case 68: Treating the obese patient—*Patricia L. Fiero, PhD & D. Walter Hiott, MD* • **77**
Case 69: Stress management—*Patricia L. Fiero, PhD & D. Walter Hiott, MD* • **78**

Case 70: **Anxiety due to a general medical condition**—*D. Walter Hiott, MD* • **79**
Case 71: **Alcohol-related irritability syndromes**—*D. Walter Hiott, MD* • **80**
Case 72: **Organic mental disorder**—*D. Walter Hiott, MD* • **81**
Case 73: **Burning pain**—*Jerome E. Kurent, MD* • **82**
Case 74: **Pain management in a geriatric patient**—*Jerome E. Kurent, MD, MPH* • **83**
Case 75: **Acute confusion in a patient with dementia**—*Jerome E. Kurent, MD, MPH* • **84**

SECTION 3: NEUROLOGY • 85

Case 76: **Weak, painful legs**—*Timothy D. Carter, MD* • **86**
Case 77: **A child with difficulty speaking**—*Timothy D. Carter, MD* • **87**
Case 78: **Funny feelings in the abdomen, olfactory hallucinations, and confusion**—*Susan M. Brown, MD* • **88**
Case 79: **A young woman with headache**—*Susan M. Brown, MD* • **89**
Case 80: **Tremor and stiffness**—*Vanessa K. Hinson, MD* • **90**
Case 81: **Progressive weakness in a young woman**—*Jerome E. Kurent, MD, MPH* • **91**
Case 82: **A newborn with spells**—*Susan M. Brown, MD* • **92**
Case 83: **"The worst headache of my life"**—*Susan M. Brown, MD* • **93**
Case 84: **Double vision**—*Timothy D. Carter, MD* • **94**
Case 85: **A 17-year-old with epilepsy and prolonged seizures**—*Susan M. Brown, MD* • **95**
Case 86: **Acute right hemiparesis**—*Timothy D. Carter, MD* • **96**
Case 87: **Back pain**—*Timothy D. Carter, MD* • **97**
Case 88: **A young woman with tremor and personality change**—*Vanessa K. Hinson, MD* • **98**
Case 89: **Severe, nightly headaches**—*Susan M. Brown, MD* • **99**
Case 90: **Transient left-sided weakness in an elderly male**—*Timothy D. Carter, MD* • **100**
Case 91: **Memory loss**—*Timothy D. Carter, MD* • **101**
Case 92: **An elderly gentleman with numbness in his feet**—*Jerome E. Kurent, MD, MPH* • **102**
Case 93: **An alcoholic with seizures**—*Susan M. Brown, MD* • **103**
Case 94: **An elderly woman with new headaches**—*Timothy D. Carter, MD* • **104**
Case 95: **Acute leg weakness in a transplant patient**—*Timothy D. Carter, MD* • **105**
Case 96: **Hand tremor in an elderly man**—*Vanessa K. Hinson, MD* • **106**
Case 97: **Altered mental status**—*Timothy D. Carter, MD* • **107**
Case 98: **Difficulty walking**—*Timothy D. Carter, MD* • **108**
Case 99: **Chronic, progressive weakness**—*Jerome E. Kurent, MD, MPH* • **109**
Case 100: **Acute collapse of a middle-aged man**—*Timothy D. Carter, MD* • **110**

Contributors

Susan M. Brown, MD
Fellow, Department of Neurology
Medical University of South Carolina
Charleston, South Carolina

Timothy D. Carter, MD
Associate Professor of Neurology
Neurology Residency Program Director
Clinical Neurophysiology Fellowship Director
Medical University of South Carolina
Charleston, South Carolina

Michael A. de Arellano, PhD
Research Assistant Professor
Clinical Psychologist
Medical University of South Carolina
Charleston, South Carolina

Mary C. Fields, MD
Fellow, Child and Adolescent Psychiatry
Department of Psychiatry
Medical University of South Carolina
Charleston, South Carolina

Patricia L. Fiero, PhD
Assistant Professor
Clinical Psychologist
Department of Psychiatry & Behavioral Sciences
Medical University of South Carolina
Charleston, South Carolina

Douglas E. Halbert, MD
Clinical Instructor in Pediatrics
The Medical University of South Carolina
Charleston, South Carolina

Vanessa K. Hinson, MD, PhD
Fellow, Section of Movement Disorders
Department of Neurological Sciences
Rush-Presbyterian-St. Luke's Medical Center
Rush University
Chicago, Illinois

D. Walter Hiott, MD
Assistant Professor of Psychiatry
Medical University of South Carolina
Attending Psychiatrist
Ralph H. Johnson VA Medical Center
Charleston, South Carolina

Janice D. Key, MD
Associate Professor of Pediatrics
Director of Adolescent Medicine
Medical University of South Carolina
Charleston, South Carolina

Matthew S. Koval, MD
Assistant Professor of Psychiatry
Medical University of South Carolina
Attending Psychiatrist
Institute of Psychiatry
Charleston, South Carolina

Jerome E. Kurent, MD, MPH
Associate Professor of Medicine, Neurology
 and Psychiatry
Medical University of South Carolina
Attending, Department of Medicine and Department
 of Neurology
Medical University Hospital
Charleston, South Carolina

Valerie M. Panzarino, MD
Assistant Professor of Pediatrics
Medical University of South Carolina
Charleston, South Carolina

Tina B. Stewart, MD
Clinical Instructor in Pediatrics
The Medical University of South Carolina
Charleston, South Carolina

Himanshu P. Upadhyaya, MBBS, MS
Assistant Professor, Psychiatry and Behavioral Sciences
Medical University of South Carolina
Institute of Psychiatry
Charleston, South Carolina

Jessica A. Whiteley, PhD
Brown Medical School Post Doctoral Fellow
Brown Medical School/The Miriam Hospital
Providence, Rhode Island

Reviewers

Bhushan S. Agharkar, MD
Resident, Department of Psychiatry and Behavioral Sciences
Emory University
Atlanta, Georgia

Carolyn J. Baxter, MD
Resident in Psychiatry
The University of Oklahoma Health Sciences Center
Tulsa, Oklahoma

Jill Breen, MD
Resident
University of Colorado Health Sciences Center
Denver, Colorado

Arun Chopra, MD
Pediatric Resident
Children's National Medical Center
Washington, DC

Scott O. Guthrie, MD
Senior Pediatric Resident
University of Tennessee College of Medicine— Chattanooga Unit
Chattanooga, Tennessee

Jennifer Heidmann, MD
Resident, Primary Care Internal Medicine
University of California, San Francisco
San Francisco, California

Craig E. Hou, MD
Resident, Department of Neurology
Washington University School of Medicine
St. Louis, Missouri

Paul V. Kotzampaltiris, MD
Chief Resident of Pediatrics
Newark's Beth Israel Medical Center
Newark, New Jersey

Leland E. Lim, MD, PhD
Resident, Department of Neurology
Stanford University
Stanford, California

Tara Miller, MD
Resident
Baylor College of Medicine
Houston, Texas

Benjamin O'Brien, MD
Resident Physician
University of Oklahoma—Tulsa
Tulsa, Oklahoma

Robert O'Brien, MD
Chief Psychiatry Resident
Northwestern Memorial Hospital
Chicago, Illinois

Sarah Schillie, MD
Resident Physician
Pennsylvania State University
Hershey, Pennsylvania

Julie Seibert, MD
Resident
University of Colorado
Denver, Colorado

David Weisman, MD
Neurology Resident
Yale University
New Haven, Connecticut

Preface

The *SleepWell Review* series is a **review for the National Board examinations,** compiled for students and residents taking parts 2 and 3 as well as international medical graduates. It is also **suitable for recertification exams in family medicine and state licensure exams.**

In the three volumes, we have attempted to cover all of the topics that you will encounter on the exams. The series differs from many practice tests, as we provide a brief discussion of the questions and answers. The emphasis is on "brief," and we do not pretend that the discussions provide a thorough review—you do not have time for that. Rather, the short explanations will remind you of the concept(s) that the board examiner wants you to know. Understand that clinical issue and you will be able to handle related questions.

Many of you will use this review as a study guide as you begin preparing for the boards. For the brave soul who decides not to study, it would be a suitable one-shot review. For most of you, we suggest using it just before the exam. After studying for months, you are burned out and cannot memorize another table or list of facts. So what do you do in the last week? Here is our best advice: go to the gym every day, get to bed early, and breeze through these sample questions with their short explanations. **Use these books** as your last study exercise, and **you will sleep well the night before the boards.**

We welcome feedback and suggestions you may have on this book or any in the new *SleepWell Review* series. Send to blue@blacksci.com.

Section 1

Pediatrics

Douglas E. Halbert, MD
Janice D. Key, MD
Valerie M. Panzarino, MD
Tina B. Stewart, MD

INFANT WITH TACHYPNEA

CASE PRESENTATION

A 5-day-old female infant presents to the emergency department with a history of poor feeding, lethargy, and tachypnea. She was born at 39 weeks gestation, with an uncomplicated vaginal delivery, and weighed 7 lbs. 5 oz. at birth. A I/VI murmur was noted in the nursery. The patient was discharged home at 48 hours of life. The baby's feedings have progressively declined until she can now only take approximately half of an ounce per feeding. Rapid breathing, wheezing, and grunting were noted by the mother during the last feeding. Physical exam is significant for a tachypneic infant with diffuse wheezes upon auscultation, hepatomegaly, delayed capillary refill, and femoral pulses that are decreased and delayed in comparison to the brachial pulses. No murmur is noted.

1. The most likely cause for the tachypnea and wheezing in this patient is:
   A. Congestive heart failure
   B. Asthma
   C. Aspiration of formula
   D. Early presentation of cystic fibrosis
   E. Tracheomalacia

2. The first thing that should be done in the emergency department is:
   A. Chest radiograph to determine the cause of the breathing problems
   B. Notify the respiratory therapist to give a treatment of albuterol
   C. Assess the patient's airway and breathing
   D. Get a better history of the feeding problems from the parents
   E. Obtain a measurement of percutaneous oxygen saturation

3. The cause of the decreased and delayed femoral pulses is most likely:
   A. Patent ductus arteriosus
   B. Shock
   C. Coarctation of the aorta
   D. Decreased/delayed femoral pulses present in all infants
   E. Aortic regurgitation

4. Chest radiograph in adolescents with this condition may reveal:
   A. A "boot shaped" heart
   B. A heart with the appearance of "an egg on a string"
   C. Rib notching
   D. Right upper lobe infiltrate
   E. Cardiomegaly

COMMENT

Coarctation of the aorta • Coarctation of the aorta accounts for 5 to 8% of congenital heart defects. It may occur alone or in combination with other defects such as bicuspid aortic valve, ventricular septal defect, patent ductus arteriosus, aortic stenosis, or mitral valve dysfunction. In fact, the initial murmur in this case may have indicated a patent ductus arteriosus, providing adequate blood flow past the coarctation until closure of the ductus after birth. Coarctation is often associated with Turner syndrome. Coarctation of the aorta causes increased afterload on the left ventricle. The closure of the ductus arteriosus may cause an acute onset of increased afterload in the neonate with severe coarctation. The patient may present in congestive heart failure.

Decreased femoral pulses • The characteristic finding on physical exam of patients with coarctation of the aorta is a delayed or decreased femoral pulse in relation to the brachial pulse. Four extremity blood pressures may be helpful, however, they are not always reliable in making the diagnosis. In coarctation of the aorta, the blood pressure in the lower extremities may be significantly lower than in the upper extremities, with a 10 to 20 mmHg difference between the two.

Feeding difficulties • Feeding difficulties in infants are common complaints to pediatricians. Feeding is one of the most energy-consumptive processes that an infant undertakes. Causes of decreased feeding may range from physiologic reflux to neonatal sepsis. This child presents with signs of significant respiratory compromise during feeding including grunting, tachypnea, and wheezing. Signs such as these should not be ignored.

Management • The ABCs (airway, breathing, and circulation) are almost always the correct answer for questions dealing with initial management of a patient. Also, please note that any infant who presents in shock should be evaluated and treated for sepsis. Patients with heart lesions may present due to exacerbation of their condition by a secondary factor such as sepsis.

Radiography • Rib notching is a late finding in patients with coarctation of the aorta. It is due to collateral circulation via enlarged intercostal vessels. The "egg on the string" appearance is found in transposition of the great vessels and not in patients with coarctation of the aorta. Likewise, "the boot shaped heart" is found in patients with tetralogy of Fallot. Right upper lobe infiltrate is sometimes found in patients with a history of aspiration pneumonia.

Answers • 1-A 2-C 3-C 4-C

CASE PRESENTATION

An 18-month-old boy is brought in to the emergency department at midnight with the chief complaint of "severe cough." The father notes that the cough developed after several days of runny nose, low-grade fever, and decreased eating. The father noticed that the boy has been eating less and he thinks that his child's throat may be sore. The cough has been getting worse each night for the past several nights. Tonight his cough was much worse but surprisingly improved on the ride into the emergency department. The patient's immunizations are up to date. On physical exam, the patient is noted to have inspiratory stridor that becomes worse when upset and a loud "barky" cough. He is tachypneic and in mild respiratory distress.

1. Of the following, which is the most likely etiologic agent for this disease process?
    A. Respiratory syncytial virus
    B. *Bordetella pertussis*
    C. *Moraxella catarrhalis*
    D. Parainfluenza virus
    E. *Haemophilus influenza* type b

2. What radiographic finding is characteristic of this disease?
    A. "Thumb sign"
    B. "Steeple sign"
    C. Right upper lobe consolidation
    D. "Boot shaped heart"
    E. Atelectasis

3. Treatment may include:
    A. Erythromycin
    B. Dexamethasone
    C. Diruretics
    D. Prophylactic intubation in the emergency department
    E. Vaccination

COMMENT

Croup • The patient described has croup or laryngotracheobronchitis, a common illness in children between the ages of 3 months and 3 years, with a mean age of 18 months. The majority of cases are caused by parainfluenza viruses (types 1, 2, and 3). Other pathogens that may cause croup include influenza, respiratory syncytial virus, and *Moraxella catarrhalis*. Croup usually occurs in the winter months, generally from October to April. Croup must be distinguished from epiglottitis, an acute, life-threatening obstruction of the upper airway due to infection and edema of the epiglottis. With vaccination against *Haemophilus influenzae*, this condition is much less common but it still must be considered in children presenting with upper airway obstruction as the clinical approach is entirely different. Children with epiglottitis must be kept comfortable with no intervention to cause worsened airway obstruction while arrangements are made to secure the airway in a controlled environment, usually the operating room.

Course • Symptoms of croup are preceded by a prodrome of mild upper respiratory tract infection with rhinorrhea, cough, low-grade fever, and occasionally sore throat. The patient subsequently develops a "barky" or "seal-like" cough and stridor that typically is worse at night or with agitation and may improve in cool moist air.

Radiography • The characteristic finding in croup on anterior posterior radiographic examination of the chest and lower airway is the "steeple sign," pointed narrowing of the superior trachea due to inflammation of the subglottic area. The "thumb sign," a thickened edge of the epiglottis when seen on lateral neck radiogram, is associated with epiglottitis. The "boot shaped" heart is associated with tetralogy of Fallot.

Therapy • Most cases of croup improve with mist humidification alone. Racemic epinephrine may be necessary if the patient does not respond to mist, however rebound symptoms may occur with worsened respiratory distress. Therefore any patient given racemic epinephrine should not be sent home from the emergency room until they have been observed for at least four hours to assess for rebound edema. Usually patients who require a dose of racemic epinephrine and definitely those who require two or more doses are admitted to the hospital. Dexamethasone is helpful in severe cases to reduce inflammation of the airway, with improvement generally occurring about six hours after administration. Intubation is reserved for severe cases and should only be performed in a very controlled environment such as an operating room by anesthesiologists.

Answers • 1-D 2-B 3-B

TODDLER WITH RECURRENT COUGH

CASE PRESENTATION

A 12-month-old African-American girl comes to see you for her one-year routine health maintenance visit. On review of her past history, you note that she has had recurrent coughing episodes and two episodes of pneumonia. Her birth history is significant for having had a meconium ileus as a newborn. There is no family history of similar illnesses. According to her mother, "She always seems to be sick." She has been to the emergency department on several occasions and her mother is concerned because "Nobody can figure out what is wrong with her." Upon further review of her case, you note that her immunizations are up to date including the pneumococcal vaccine. Her mother is also concerned that she is small for her age despite having an excellent appetite. Mom does note that the patient's stools are malodorous. On physical examination her weight is 7 kg (5%), length 71 cm (10%), and head circumference 45 cm (25%). The rest of her physical examination is normal.

1. Which test would be the most helpful in making the diagnosis in this case?
   A. pH probe
   B. DNA analysis for the deletion at position 508 in the CF gene
   C. Sweat chloride
   D. Immunoglobulin levels
   E. Bronchial aspirate

2. Which of the following is not associated with the disease?
   A. Jaundice
   B. Gallstones
   C. Failure to thrive
   D. Nasal polyps
   E. Recurrent pneumonia
   F. All of the above are associated with the disease

3. Which of the following organisms is least likely to colonize the lungs of older children and adolescents with this disease?
   A. *Haemophilus influenzae*
   B. *Pseudomonas aeruginosa*
   C. *Staphylococcus aureus*
   D. *Burkholderia cepacia*
   E. *Streptococcus pneumoniae*

COMMENT

Cystic fibrosis • This child's presentation is typical of cystic fibrosis (CF). While CF is more common in Caucasians than African-Americans, with an incidence among Caucasians of approximately 1 in 2500 live births and among African-Americans, 1 in 17,000 live births, it is still important to always consider the diagnosis. Conditions suggestive of cystic fibrosis in this case include meconium ileus at birth, the history of malodorous stools due to the malabsorption caused by pancreatic insufficiency, recurrent pneumonia, and failure to thrive. Other clinical manifestations of cystic fibrosis include nasal polyps, recurrent sinusitis, cholelithiasis, biliary obstruction and ultimately cirrhosis, pancreatitis, diabetes mellitus, intestinal obstruction, bronchiectasis, and hemoptysis.

Etiology • CF is caused by several distinct defects in the enzyme responsible for pumping chloride through the transmembrane channel, resulting in altered and thickened secretions from several organs including the lungs, pancreas, and sweat glands. The most common gene causing CF, $\Delta 508$, a deletion in the CF gene at position 508 of the long arm of chromosome 7, is present in 70% of Caucasians with CF but is less common in African-Americans. Therefore, the most sensitive test in this case may be the sweat chloride test. False positives in the sweat chloride test in children are rare but may be due to glycogen storage diseases, hypothyroidism, or severe malnutrition.

Infections • Children with CF are living much longer with advancement in antibiotics, pancreatic enzyme replacement, and interventions to decrease pulmonary complications. As patients are treated with multiple antibiotics and develop chronic lung disease they tend to become colonized with *Staphylococcus aureus* and *Pseudomonas aeruginosa*, often with these organisms developing resistance to the antibiotics that have been used for treatment. Common organisms in the respiratory tract also include the flora seen in healthy children such as *Streptococcus pneumoniae* and nontypable *Haemophilus influenzae*. *Burkholderia cepacia* is an infrequent organism in CF patients, usually acquired later in older patients with severe illness.

Answers • 1-C 2-F 3-D

CASE PRESENTATION

A 5-year-old female is seen for a chief complaint of "worsening rash." The patient was diagnosed with a urinary tract infection about eight days ago and started on trimethoprim sulfamethoxazole. Five days after starting the medication, the patient developed "flu-like" symptoms consisting of fever, cough, sore throat, and itchy, burning eyes. Two days later a rash appeared and the patient complained of increasing oral pain and was not able to swallow her secretions. Since then the rash has gradually spread. On physical exam, the patient has extensive macular erythematous target lesions–many of which are becoming confluent. Her eye exam is significant for erythematous conjunctiva with edema and tearing.

1. What is the most likely diagnosis?
   A. Pityriasis rosea
   B. Parvovirus B19 infection
   C. Erythema multiforme minor
   D. Stevens-Johnson syndrome
   E. Gram negative sepsis

2. The most appropriate treatment would include which of the following?
   A. Start an aminoglycoside for improved bacterial coverage
   B. Increase the dose of the trimethoprim-sulfamethoxazole due to the emergence of resistant organisms
   C. Continue the trimethoprim-sulfamethoxazole to fully treat the urinary tract infection
   D. Discontinue the trimethoprim-sulfamethoxazole
   E. Treat with a short course of corticosteroids

3. The most likely prognosis for this patient is:
   A. The risk of mortality is significant and the patient may have recurrence of the disease in the future
   B. The disease will respond well to outpatient treatment and the patient will have no sequelae
   C. The symptoms may worsen, requiring hospitalization, but will have no sequelae
   D. The disease is self-limited and the patient will improve with minimal intervention
   E. The patient will probably develop an autoimmune illness in the future

COMMENT

Erythema multiforme • Erythema multiforme (EM) is a spectrum of diseases that include erythema multiforme minor, erythema multiforme major (also known as Stevens-Johnson syndrome), and possibly toxic epidermal necrolysis. EM is often associated with a medication but may also be associated with preceding infections (such as mycoplasma pneumonia), or may be idiopathic.

Prognosis • The difference between EM minor, EM major, and toxic epidermal necrolysis is the severity of illness. EM minor is generally a self limited disease with low morbidity, affecting mainly the skin with no more than one mucosal surface involved. EM major is more severe and involves two or more mucous membranes. It may also affect internal organs and causes more systemic symptoms. There is a mortality rate of up to 10% with EM major. Toxic epidermal necrolysis is viewed by some as a more severe case of EM while others view it as a separate disease entity.

Treatment • An important step in treating the disease is to remove the offending agent–stop using the causative drug or treat underlying disease. Supportive care is paramount with aggressive fluid management and treatment of secondary infection. Ophthalmology consultation should be requested to carefully examine and follow patients as significant ocular sequel may occur. Corticosteroid use is controversial.

Answers • 1-D 2-D 3-A

PRESCHOOL CHILD WITH A SEIZURE

● CASE PRESENTATION

A 3-year-old white male with no prior medical problems experiences a five-minute generalized tonic-clonic seizure. He is brought to the emergency room and seems somewhat tired initially but then is active and playful. His initial temperature is 103 degrees Fahrenheit rectally. The parents report that the patient is in daycare and has had upper respiratory infection symptoms for the past two days. On physical exam, no focal neurological deficits can be found.

1. The fact that the seizure was generalized and tonic-clonic is:
   A. Reassuring since it indicates that there was no particular focus
   B. Concerning since it indicates that this patient most likely has meningitis
   C. Concerning since this patient is in daycare and may be infected with a more resistant organism
   D. Not helpful diagnostically
   E. Makes a recurrence less likely

2. The history of upper respiratory infection symptoms is useful in this case because:
   A. It indicates that this patient has bacterial sinusitis which has resulted in a brain abscess
   B. It is the most likely source for this patient's fever
   C. This patient should be placed in an isolation room to prevent further spread of the organism
   D. Upper respiratory infections often cause seizures in children in this age group
   E. It eliminates the possibility of meningitis

3. The duration of the seizure indicates:
   A. That this is most likely a benign seizure
   B. Nothing–the duration is not helpful diagnostically or prognostically
   C. That this patient is at great risk for subsequent seizures and epilepsy
   D. That this patient may have suffered permanent brain damage from the seizure
   E. The patient is in status epilepticus

4. Therapy for this patient at this point should include:
   A. Intravenous antibiotics
   B. Admission to the hospital and close observation
   C. Oral antibiotics
   D. Antiepileptic medications
   E. None of the above

● COMMENT

Febrile seizures • Febrile seizures are fairly common occurrences during childhood, usually occurring in children with a rapidly rising fever. In the United States, between 2 and 4% of children will have a febrile seizure by their fifth birthday. Febrile seizures generally occur in children who are between 6 months of age and 4 years of age. The majority of affected children will have only one seizure episode although some will have two or three febrile seizures during childhood. It is thought that kids in this age group may have a lower seizure threshold. Viral illnesses are the main cause of febrile seizures. Shigella gastroenteritis and human herpes simplex virus 6 induced roseola are commonly associated with febrile seizures.

Types • Febrile seizures are classified into two types. Simple febrile seizures last less than 15 minutes and are generalized. Complex febrile seizures are prolonged, recur more than once in a 24-hour period, are focal/unilateral, or are followed by transient (Todd's) paralysis.

Risk factors • Risk factors for febrile seizure recurrence include children who have had more than one seizure, have a first febrile seizure before 6 months of age, have a family history of a febrile seizure, or have complex febrile seizures. The risk for developing epilepsy is only slightly higher in comparison with the rate of the general population: 1% versus 0.5%.

Lab studies/Imaging studies • Routine laboratory studies are generally not necessary unless the etiology of the fever is unknown. Electrolytes are usually not helpful. A CT scan of the brain is usually not required for patients with simple febrile seizures. Because fevers and seizures are associated with meningitis, one should have a low threshold for performing a lumbar puncture, especially in younger children or in patients who are already on antibiotic therapy, as the clinical findings of meningitis are more subtle in these patients.

Treatment • Antiepileptic medications are not necessary for this patient and are generally not used to prevent further febrile seizures. Antipyretics are often used to relieve discomfort but do not seem to reduce the recurrence of febrile seizures. Hospital admission for simple febrile seizures is usually not necessary. Parents should be educated about what to do if the patient has another seizure.

Answers • 1-A 2-B 3-A 4-E

CASE PRESENTATION

A 15-year-old high school athlete presents with increasing fatigue and weakness in the lower extremities over the last week. He has noticed that he is more "clumsy" than usual and often finds himself tripping unexpectedly. The patient is concerned that his weakness has been getting worse. He has noticed a painful tingling sensation in his lower extremities at times. He will be starting the sports season in several weeks and wonders if these symptoms are just his imagination and due to stress. He notes that several weeks ago, he had a nonspecific illness that resolved without treatment. On physical exam, the patient is areflexic and has significant weakness in the lower extremities. His gait is somewhat ataxic.

1. This patient is most likely suffering from:
   A. Severe hypothyroidism
   B. Multiple sclerosis
   C. Guillain-Barré syndrome
   D. Lyme disease
   E. Muscular dystrophy

2. Diagnosis is best confirmed by which of the following tests:
   A. Thyroid function testing
   B. Thorough skin exam
   C. Nerve conduction studies
   D. Serum titers
   E. MRI

3. The weakness in this disease generally:
   A. Occurs asymmetrically
   B. Occurs symmetrically
   C. Spares the diaphragm
   D. Occurs permanently
   E. Presents in a descending pattern

COMMENT

Guillain-Barré syndrome • Guillain-Barré syndrome (GBS) is a demyelinating polyneuropathy presenting as a progressive disorder characterized by ascending motor weakness, hyporeflexia, and paresthesias. The weakness may have a sudden onset but may progress over hours or several weeks. Weakness is generally symmetric. Early recognition of this disorder is important due to the risk of respiratory muscle paralysis and hypoventilation.

Etiology • The cause of this disease is not completely understood. It is believed to be an autoimmune disease that causes demyelination of peripheral nerves and spinal roots. Two-thirds of patients have had an antecedent infection. These are generally gastrointestinal or respiratory infections. GBS has also very rarely been associated with some immunizations. Children are generally at lower risk for this disease than are adults. Due to the great strides in preventing disease from poliomyelitis, this disease is now the leading cause of acute non-traumatic paralysis in most parts of the world.

Presentation and diagnosis • The most striking observation on physical examination is the weakness in the lower extremities. Patients will eventually become nonambulatory. Weakness in the deltoid and biceps muscle may precede hypoventilation as the paralysis ascends. Cranial nerves may also be involved and can cause respiratory difficulties due to vocal cord or laryngeal muscle weakness. Cerebral spinal fluid studies are necessary to confirm the diagnosis, with significantly elevated protein levels. Nerve conduction studies demonstrate slowed conduction but these findings may lag behind clinical findings. MRI with gadolinium usually shows enhancement of cauda equina nerve roots.

Therapy and prognosis • Plasma exchange and serum immunoglobulin therapy may shorten recovery time. Prevention of complications such as hypoventilation is critical for these patients. Full recovery occurs in the majority of cases although permanent sequelae may result from GBS.

Answers • 1-C 2-C 3-B

CASE PRESENTATION

A 14-year-old boy comes to your office complaining of a cough for nine days. His symptoms have gradually worsened with rhinorrhea, sore throat, fever, headache, and malaise. He has missed the last four days of school. Over the past several days, the fever and cough have worsened. He states that he feels very mildly short of breath if he tries to go up the stairs. His cough has been productive of white sputum. On physical examination, he has a temperature of 101.5 degrees Fahrenheit orally and a respiratory rate of 25 breaths per minute. Fine crackles and wheezes are heard bilaterally upon auscultation of the patient's chest.

1. The most likely organism causing this patient's pneumonia is:
   A. *Streptococcus pneumoniae*
   B. *Haemophilus influenzae*
   C. *Moraxella catarrhalis*
   D. *Mycoplasma pneumoniae*
   E. *Pneumocystis carinii*

2. Which antibiotic would be most beneficial in the treatment of this patient's disease?
   A. Amoxicillin
   B. Ceftriaxone
   C. Azithromycin
   D. Penicillin
   E. Sulfonamides

3. *Mycoplasma pneumoniae* infection may be associated with:
   A. Hemolytic anemia
   B. Increased atypical lymphocytes (Downy cells)
   C. Polycythemia
   D. Chronic respiratory acidosis
   E. Septic arthritis

COMMENT

Mycoplasma pneumonia • Mycoplasma pneumonia, "atypical pneumonia," is the most common cause of pneumonia in school-age children and adolescents. The initial symptoms of infection are nonspecific and more gradual in onset than in other forms of bacterial pneumonia. Disease progresses from the upper respiratory tract and proceeds to the lower respiratory tract. A productive cough is common but not always present and is not as severe as in pneumonias caused by other pathogens such with *Streptococcus pneumoniae*. Diffuse wheezes and crackles are often found rather than distinct rales. *Streptococcus pneumoniae*, *Haemophilus pneumoniae* (especially in unimmunized children), *Chlamydia pneumoniae* and *Moraxella catarrhalis* are all important causes of pneumonia as well as other diseases such as otitis media and sinusitis in children and adolescents. *Pneumocystis carinii* usually only causes disease in immunocompromised patients, such as patients with AIDS.

Diagnosis • The diagnosis is usually clinical. Chest x-rays are variable and may be entirely normal. Bacterial culture is of limited use because isolation takes between 7 and 21 days. While nonspecific, coagulation of red blood cells with cold agglutinins is positive in 50% of adolescents with atypical pneumonia. This effect of reversible agglutination with cold temperature is caused by elevated IgM antibodies that are directed toward certain types of red blood cells.

Therapy and prognosis • Mycoplasma pneumonia is best treated with a macrolide antibiotic such as erythromycin, clarithromycin, or azithromycin, all of which are equally effective although the newer macrolides, such as azithromycin, have fewer side effects. Tetracyclines are also effective for mycoplasma pneumonia. Penicillins and other similar antibiotics are not effective as *Mycoplasma pneumoniae* does not have a cell wall. When the treatment is delayed beyond the initial infection, antibiotic therapy may have little impact on the prolonged course of cough and wheezing, symptoms that persist while the damaged respiratory lining slowly regenerates motile cilia. While usually a mild illness, mycoplasma infection may cause a wide range of other clinical problems including hemolytic anemia, arthritis, rash, neurological complications, erythema multiforme and Stevens-Johnson syndrome. These symptoms in diffuse sites, such as arthritis and meningitis, are secondary to an immune response rather than direct infection of those sites.

Answers • 1-D 2-C 3-A

CASE PRESENTATION

A 2-year-old African-American boy presents with a fever and a history of pulling at his right ear. His mother has been treating him with acetaminophen but he is still somewhat irritable. He has had two prior episodes of ear infections in the past year. He is in daycare. His grandparents live with him and his mother and they smoke, but only outside the house. On physical examination, he is nontoxic, well hydrated and has a bulging, erythematous right tympanic membrane.

1. Which of the following organisms is not a common pathogen for acute otitis media?
   A. *Streptoccoccus pneumoniae*
   B. *Haemophilus influenzae* type B
   C. *Moraxella catarrhalis*
   D. *Streptococcus pyogenes*
   E. Adenovirus

2. Risk factors for otitis media include:
   A. Prior otitis media
   B. Family history of frequent otitis media
   C. Exposure to tobacco smoke
   D. Down syndrome
   E. All of the above

3. The fact that this child is in daycare is important because:
   A. His ear infection is more likely to be viral due to the constant exposure to other children
   B. Children in daycare tend to have fewer resistant bacterial infections
   C. Daycare attendance is not a risk factor for developing otitis media
   D. Daycare attendance increases the risk of a resistant bacterial infection
   E. His ear infection is more likely to be bacterial due to the constant exposure to other children

4. Risk factors for recurrent otitis media include:
   A. Inadequate immunization
   B. Bottle feeding
   C. Household pets
   D. Cold weather
   E. Failure to thrive

5. If this patient developed postauricular swelling or erythema and displacement of the pinna, what complication should you be concerned about?
   A. Meningitis
   B. Perforation of the tympanic membrane
   C. Localized lymphadenitis
   D. Mastoiditis
   E. Brain abscess

COMMENT

Otitis media • Acute otitis media is an infection of the middle ear characterized by bulging and erythema of the tympanic membrane, otalgia, fever, irritability, and decreased hearing. Infection can be either viral or bacterial. The three most common bacterial pathogens include *Streptococcus pneumoniae*, *Haemophilus influenzae* (nontypeable), and *Moraxella catarrhalis*. The overall incidence of *Haemophilus influenza* type B has been drastically reduced by the Hib vaccine and *Haemophilus influenza* type B is no longer a common pathogen in acute otitis media. The new use of seven valent pneumococcal vaccine has been shown to decrease the incidence of otitis media but certainly does not eliminate the disease as it is caused by many other organisms and additional strains of pneumococcus.

Risk factors • Risk factors for otitis media include prior otitis media, male gender, tobacco smoke exposure, bottle feeding/propping, genetic predisposition, and craniofacial abnormalities such as in Down syndrome or cleft palate. Children who attend daycare and children from lower socioeconomic status families have a higher incidence of otitis media. Daycare attendance is also associated with strains of bacteria that may be higher in resistance to some of the antibiotics commonly used in the treatment of otitis media.

Treatment • Because differentiation of viral otitis media from bacterial otitis media is not possible with most patients, treatment includes antibiotics that will be effective against the common pathogens, such as amoxicillin. High-dose amoxicillin should be considered in areas or situations where resistant *Streptococcus pneumoniae* is suspected. Other antibiotic alternatives include amoxicillin with clavulanic acid, azithromycin, and certain cephalosporins. Analgesics and antipyretics are helpful in alleviating discomfort. Treatment should also address the underlying risk factors for an individual patient to prevent recurrence. Myringotomy tubes should be considered for children with recurrent infection or persistent serous otitis despite all medical interventions.

Mastoiditis • Extension of bacterial infection from the middle ear into the mastoid is an increasingly rare but serious complication, as the mastoid air cells communicate with the middle ear. Clinical findings that indicate mastoiditis include postauricular swelling or erythema and outward displacement of the pinna. When it occurs, mastoiditis requires more intensive antibiotic therapy and may require surgical intervention.

Answers • 1-B 2-E 3-D 4-B 5-D

CASE PRESENTATION

A 13-year-old obese girl presents to the emergency department with a one-month history of intermittent headaches and visual changes. She notes that she has had decreased visual acuity and occasional "double vision." She had her first menstrual period approximately two months ago and was started on a medication for her acne by her primary care doctor. Her schoolteacher instructed her to "see an eye doctor" because of the headaches and vision problems. The doctor dilated her pupils and, after performing a fundic examination that revealed papilledema, he referred her to the emergency department for further evaluation.

1. What findings on magnetic resonance imaging of the head would be consistent with pseudotumor cerebri?
   A. Tumor obstructing the third ventricle
   B. Enlarged ventricles
   C. White matter changes of various ages
   D. Normal appearance of brain and ventricles
   E. Hemorrhage

2. What is the most likely cause of this patient's "double vision?"
   A. Bilateral optic nerve atrophy
   B. Cranial nerve IV palsy
   C. Cranial nerve VI palsy
   D. Tumor compressing the optic chiasm
   E. Macular degeneration

3. Which of the following are risk factors for developing pseudotumor cerebri?
   A. Female gender
   B. Obesity
   C. Tetracycline
   D. Adolescent or young adult
   E. All of the above are risk factors

4. Therapy of this disorder would not include which of the following?
   A. Aetazolamide therapy
   B. Emergent lumbar puncture
   C. Ventriculoperitoneal shunting
   D. Serial lumbar punctures
   E. Ophthalmology follow-up

COMMENT

Pseudotumor cerebri • Pseudotumor cerebri, as implied by its name, presents with increased intracranial pressure but without a cause such as a tumor. It has historically also been called benign intracranial hypertension as well as idiopathic intracranial hypertension. The etiology of the increased intracranial pressure is still not completely understood. Symptoms are related to the elevated intracranial pressure and include: a nonspecific headache, diplopia due to sixth cranial nerve palsy, photophobia, and visual disturbances due to papilledema. Papilledema, present in the majority of patients, may cause progressive vision loss in one or both eyes, starting in the nasal inferior quadrant followed by loss of central visual field. A rare complication of sudden visual loss may occur due to intraocular hemorrhage resulting from revascularization related to the chronic papilledema.

Risk factors • Epidemiologic studies have shown that female gender, obesity, menstrual irregularity, recent weight gain, reproductive age-group, and certain medications are all risk factors for pseudotumor cerebri. Medications associated with pseudotumor may include: vitamin A (particularly in excessive doses), growth hormone, tetracycline, minocycline, corticosteroids, isotretinoin, trimethoprim-sulfamethoxazole, and lithium.

Diagnosis • Prior to performing a lumbar puncture to measure intracranial pressure, an imaging study (computer tomography scan or magnetic resonance imaging) should be obtained to rule out other causes of increased headache and intracranial pressure such as hydrocephalus, intracranial mass or tumor, meningeal inflammation or disease, or dural venous sinus thrombosis. Lumbar puncture in some of these other conditions may result in rapid cerebral herniation and even death. When the lumbar puncture is performed, the opening pressure must be obtained in addition to other routine studies of the spinal fluid: cell count and differential, total protein, glucose, and culture.

Therapy • The initial lumbar puncture may be helpful diagnostically as well as therapeutically as removal of spinal fluid will decrease the intracranial pressure. Occasionally patients may require additional lumbar punctures with removal of spinal fluid. Medical treatment includes acetazolamide, a carbonic anhydrase inhibitor, to decrease production of cerebral spinal fluid, in addition to elimination of associated risk factors. Severe cases may require ventriculoperitoneal shunting to control intracranial pressure or even optic nerve fenestration to prevent further optic nerve complications. Patients should be carefully monitored, including serial neuro-ophthalmologic examinations, to prevent these complications.

Answers • 1-D 2-C 3-E 4-B

CASE PRESENTATION

A 3-year-old boy has been progressively fatigued over the past week. His parents have been concerned because the patient has lost several pounds during the past several months. Today the patient's mother noticed that there was some blood on the patient's toothbrush and that he had developed "spots" on his skin. On physical examination, the boy has a fever of 102 degrees orally. He is somewhat pale and has petechiae where the blood pressure cuff compressed his arm. He has diffuse lymphadenopathy and hepatosplenomegaly.

1. The most common pediatric malignancy is:
   A. Acute myeloid leukemia (AML)
   B. Acute lymphoblastic leukemia (ALL)
   C. Hodgkin's disease
   D. Chronic myelogenous leukemia (CML)
   E. Brain tumor

2. In patients with this malignancy, an initial chest x-ray is performed to determine the presence of:
   A. Pulmonary metastases
   B. Pneumonia
   C. Heart size prior to chemotherapy
   D. Mediastinal mass
   E. Pleural effusion

3. Which of the following is not associated with tumor lysis syndrome?
   A. Hyperuricemia
   B. Hypokalemia
   C. Hypocalcemia
   D. Hyperphosphatemia
   E. Elevated creatinine

4. The overall cure rate for childhood ALL is approximately:
   A. 10%
   B. 20%
   C. 30%
   D. 50%
   E. 70%

COMMENT

Acute lymphoblastic leukemia (ALL) • ALL is the most common malignancy of childhood, accounting for one-third of all pediatric cancers, with a peak incidence at about 3 to 4 years old. Brain tumors are the most common solid malignancy of childhood. ALL is a disease caused by dysregulation of the hematopoietic cells. Leukemic cells spread throughout the body into places such as the bone marrow, thymus, liver, spleen, lymph nodes, testes, and CNS. ALL was the first childhood cancer treated with chemotherapy. From those days of experimental treatment, when ALL was a uniformly fatal illness, cure rates have improved and are now greater than 70%.

Clinical presentation and evaluation • Most patients present with a combination of signs and symptoms including pallor, bleeding, easy bruisability, weight loss, lethargy, anorexia, fever, bone pain, or joint pain. Physical examination may reveal lymphadenopathy, hepatosplenomegaly, petechiae, ecchymoses, bone tenderness, enlarged testes, or enlarged salivary glands. Laboratory studies often demonstrate effects on multiple cell lines such as anemia, abnormal white blood cell counts (either elevated or decreased), and thrombocytopenia, although a normal complete blood count does not exclude the diagnosis of leukemia. Peripheral blood smears may show lymphoblasts. Chest x-ray should be performed to look for mediastinal masses, due to lymphadenopathy, that may impinge upon the airway. Bone marrow aspirates and lumbar puncture are performed to assess extent of disease.

Tumor lysis syndrome • During initiation of chemotherapy, there may be a rapid release of intracellular contents from the leukemic cells. This release may result in hyperuricemia, hyperphosphatemia, hypocalcemia, and hyperkalemia. Renal failure may occur due to uric acid nephropathy. Close electrolyte monitoring, IV hydration, alkalinization of the urine to increase phosphate/uric acid clearance, and allopurinol are critical to prevent these complications.

Answers • 1-B 2-D 3-B 4-E

TODDLER WITH DEVELOPMENTAL DELAY

CASE PRESENTATION

An 18-month-old boy presents to your office for a well-child check. His mother is concerned about developmental problems. You decide to consider several different diagnoses.

1. Which of the following physical findings is not suggestive of cerebral palsy?
   A. Tongue thrusts
   B. Strabismus
   C. Hypertonicity
   D. Regression of motor skills
   E. Persistent primitive reflexes

2. Autism is associated with which of the following developmental problems?
   A. Clumsiness
   B. Ritualistic behavior
   C. Deafness
   D. Aggressive behavior
   E. Difficulty in separation

3. Of the developmental conditions listed below, which is not associated with language delay?
   A. Visual impairment
   B. Mental retardation
   C. Hearing impairment
   D. Environmental deprivation
   E. Autism

COMMENT

Cerebral palsy (CP) • CP is a nonprogressive disorder of movement and posture and is classified as a static encephalopathy. This definition of CP clarifies that a **regression** of motor skills is not due to CP. Losing developmental milestones is a "red flag" in pediatrics and points to different etiologies including neurodegenerative diseases. It is difficult to make the diagnosis of CP prior to 1 year of age due to the nonspecific and variable findings on physical exam. Patients often have decreased tone, increased reflexes, and difficulty with sucking and swallowing during infancy. By 12 months of age, the initial hypotonia begins developing into hypertonia. The patient can also exhibit tongue thrusts, grimacing, posturing, strabismus, persistent primitive reflexes, and increased deep tendon reflexes. Patients with CP often also have other neurologic conditions such as seizures, speech delay, abnormal vision, and mental retardation. The etiologies of CP can be divided into categories including prenatal (such as infection, genetic conditions, or placental insufficiency), perinatal (such as anoxia during delivery), and immediately postnatal (such as toxins, trauma, or infection).

Autism • Autism is in a spectrum of pervasive developmental disorders and is characterized by delayed language development and abnormal social behavior. These children have poor verbal and nonverbal communication skills, do not read other's emotions, do not share enjoyment, have poor peer relationships, have no pretend play, use echolalia, perform rituals, do not tolerate change well, and exhibit visual tracking. These children do not have any motor deficits that would be expected with clumsiness.

Language delays • Language delays are not associated with visual impairment. These children can have problems with language that requires use of visual concepts, but their overall language skills are normal. Hearing impairment, mental retardation, environmental deprivation, autism, and language disabilities are all associated with language delays.

Answers • 1-D 2-B 3-A

CASE PRESENTATION

A previously healthy 6-year-old boy presents with fatigue, easy bruising, and a petechial rash. When he brushes his teeth, he has noted some bleeding of his gums over the past several days. Upon further questioning, the patient recalls having a recent viral illness that resolved spontaneously several weeks ago. Physical exam is normal except a few nonblanching, petechial, macular lesions, less than 0.5 cm, on his lower legs. He has no lymphadenopathy or hepatosplenomegaly. A complete blood cell count reveals a low platelet count (<20,000 per cubic milliliter) but normal values in the other cell lines.

1. The low platelet count is most likely due to:
   A. Disseminated intravascular coagulation
   B. Impaired production of platelets
   C. Antibody production against the platelets
   D. Erroneous value due to lab error
   E. Congenital platelet defect

2. Bone marrow biopsy of this child would reveal:
   A. Increased numbers of blast cells
   B. Paucity of all cell lines
   C. Normal or increased number of megakaryocytes
   D. Decreased numbers of megakaryocytes
   E. Osteopetrosis

3. A peripheral blood smear would show:
   A. Large platelets
   B. Clumps of platelets
   C. Schistocytes
   D. Small platelets
   E. Hypochromic red blood cells

COMMENT

Idiopathic thrombocytopenic purpura • Acute ITP is an acquired thrombocytopenic disorder with a low platelet count, petechial rash, normal bone marrow, and no other causes of thrombocytopenia. It is caused by platelet destruction in the reticuloendothelial system due to platelet glycoprotein autoantibodies. Acute ITP is more prevalent in children younger than 10 years old. Prior viral infections may sensitize the immune system to the platelet antigens. Bone marrow biopsy, while not always indicated, would demonstrate normal or increased numbers of megakaryocytes. Platelets are larger in size on peripheral smear due to the increased destruction and larger proportion of younger platelets.

Differential diagnosis • An important differentiation from other more serious illnesses is the fact that the other cell lines are not affected in this disorder. The differential diagnosis for this thrombocytopenia is extensive. Pseudothrombocytopenia, a laboratory error when platelets are clumped due to improper collection or transport of a blood sample, results in an artificially low platelet count. Other causes of thrombocytopenia include: decreased production (malignancy, aplastic anemia, and congenital syndromes such as thrombocytopenia-absent radius (TAR) syndrome and Fanconi syndrome), increased destruction (autoimmune diseases, disseminated intravascular coagulation, or giant hemangioma), and sequestration (splenomegaly). History, physical examination, and production of other cell lines can differentiate these conditions.

Treatment • The majority of patients will recover without any treatment. There is a small risk of intracranial hemorrhage in patients with a significantly lowered platelet count. In these patients, intravenous immnoglobulin and steroids have been used. Medications that impair platelet function such as nonsteroidal anti-inflammatory medications or aspirin should be avoided. Platelet transfusions are not helpful as the circulating antibodies will rapidly destroy these platelets.

Answers • 1-C 2-C 3-A

CASE PRESENTATION

A 13-year-old girl presents with heavy, prolonged vaginal bleeding. She had menarche at age 12 and since then has had monthly vaginal bleeding with 10 to 14 days of heavy bleeding occurring every 21 to 25 days. She also complains of mild lower abdominal cramping with each episode of bleeding. She denies sexual activity. Her physical examination is normal.

1. What laboratory test is most important in the initial management of this patient?
   A. Pelvic ultrasound
   B. Follicular stimulating hormone and luteinizing hormone
   C. Hemoglobin
   D. Testing for gonorrhea and chlamydia
   E. Pregnancy test

2. What laboratory test is most likely to diagnose this patient's illness?
   A. Complete blood count and differential
   B. Factor VIII activity
   C. Estrogen level
   D. Prothrombin time and partial thromboplastin time
   E. Factor IX activity

3. What medical treatment would be most effective in minimizing her symptoms and illness?
   A. Combined oral contraceptives and iron supplement
   B. Monthly use of progesterone for 5 to 10 days and iron supplement
   C. Menstrual calendar and iron supplement
   D. Monthly use of DDAVP (desmopressin acetate)
   E. Blood transfusion

COMMENT

Menorrhagia and coagulopathy • Menorrhagia is heavy and prolonged vaginal bleeding occurring in a regular monthly cycle. Adolescent girls who present with menorrhagia since menarche often have a disorder of coagulation. This may include inherited disorders of platelet number and function, aplastic anemia, and thrombocytopenia due to bone marrow infiltration as with leukemia. However, the most common coagulopathy in these patients in von Willebrand's disease, an inherited disorder of a protein necessary for platelet adhesion and factor VIII function. Inheritance can occur as either an autosomal dominant or autosomal recessive trait and can be due to either underproduction or inactivity of the von Willebrand's protein. As this protein is involved in platelet and factor VIII function, both bleeding time and factor VIII level and function may be abnormal. Prothrombin time is normal and partial thrombopastin time is usually normal but may be slightly prolonged. Additional testing of the von Willebrand's factor antigen and activity (ristocetin cofactor) may specifically diagnose von Willebrand's disease.

Management of menorrhagia • Initial management of a patient with menorrhagia should always include evaluation of the degree of anemia as this will determine the immediate treatment, ranging from careful monitoring of the hemoglobin to iron supplementation to transfusion, and may also determine whether immediate cessation of vaginal bleeding with high-dose estrogen is necessary. Long-term management usually involves decreasing the endometrial lining and therefore the monthly withdrawal bleeding through the use of low-dose combination estrogen, progestin pills, and iron supplementation until the anemia resolves and iron stores are replenished. Emergency management of severe bleeding due to von Willebrand's disease also includes desmopressin that results in a temporary increase in release of von Willebrand's protein. Transfusion may be necessary if anemia is severe and the patient is symptomatic.

Answers • 1-C 2-B 3-A

● CASE PRESENTATION

A 5-year-old Caucasian boy presents due to the parents' concern that he is "walking funny." At first, they thought that the child was playing, but the gait has persisted and now the patient is having difficulty walking up stairs. On physical examination, the patient has proximal muscle weakness in his legs. When the patient tries to rise from the floor, he pushes on his knees in order to stand. Deep tendon reflexes are slightly decreased in the distal extremities. He is unable to jump and falls during the examination.

1. What sign is described in the vignette above? ("When the patient tries to rise from the floor, he pushes on his knees in order to stand.")
   A. Darier's sign
   B. Gowers' sign
   C. Trendelenburg's sign
   D. Trousseau's sign
   E. Normal development for a 5-year-old

2. Of the following, what laboratory test would be most helpful in establishing the diagnosis?
   A. Uric acid
   B. Calcium
   C. Creatine kinase
   D. Lactate dehydrogenase
   E. Complete blood count

3. Of the following, which gene is associated with this group of disorders?
   A. Fibrillin gene
   B. Spectrin gene
   C. Collagenase gene
   D. Dystrophin gene

4. The mechanism of inheritance for this disorder is:
   A. X-linked recessive
   B. Autosomal recessive
   C. X-linked dominant
   D. Autosomal dominant
   E. Multifactorial

● COMMENT

Muscular dystrophy (MD) • MD, an inherited, degenerative disease of skeletal muscle occurring mainly in boys, is characterized by progressive muscle weakness. The most common types of MD that present in childhood are Duchenne and Becker. Both are characterized by progressive muscle weakness, initially affecting the proximal muscles and manifesting as weakness walking up stairs and development of a waddling gait. Both occur as X-linked recessive conditions, however, they differ in clinical onset of symptoms and course, with Becker MD patients becoming symptomatic at an older age and having a more gradual decline in function. Findings on physical examination include the Gower sign (pushing on the knee to assist with standing up), muscle pseudohypertrophy (especially calves), toe walking, scoliosis, forward tilt of the pelvis with lordosis, and decreased deep tendon reflexes.

Diagnostic testing • As MD involves destruction of muscle cells, intracellular enzymes from these dying cells are increased in the serum. Creatine phosphokinase (CK) is markedly elevated in both Duchenne and Becker muscular dystrophy. Muscle biopsy demonstrates muscle degeneration and regeneration with proliferation of connective tissue and mononuclear inflammatory cell infiltrate. Genetic testing has become available with identification of the specific gene that causes muscular dystrophy, the dystrophin gene located at the Xp21 locus.

Answers • 1-B 2-C 3-D 4-A

ILLNESS IN A NEONATE

CASE PRESENTATION

An infant presents with temperature instability at 4 hours of age, requiring external warming to maintain a normal temperature. He was a full-term infant with adequate prenatal care, a negative prenatal history and normal vaginal delivery. On physical examination he is appropriate size for a full-term infant (AGA) and has a normal physical examination except slight cyanosis of his hands and feet and a delay in his capillary refill.

1. Which clinical presentation is not associated with neonatal sepsis?
   A. Respiratory distress
   B. Fever or hypothermia
   C. Apnea
   D. Poor perfusion and shock
   E. Erythema toxicum

2. Which of the following does not increase the risk of neonatal sepsis?
   A. Prematurity
   B. Female gender
   C. Chorioamnionitis
   D. Prolonged rupture of membranes
   E. Maternal fever

3. Which of the following statements is true regarding neonatal sepsis?
   A. Urine cultures obtained by bag specimens are as reliable as those obtained by suprapubic tap.
   B. A lumbar puncture should be performed only if signs of meningitis are present.
   C. Leukocytosis and not neutropenia is found in patients with neonatal sepsis.
   D. An increased ratio of immature neutrophils to total neutrophils may be found in neonatal sepsis.
   E. Chest radiographs are infrequently obtained in the evaluation of neonatal sepsis.

4. The most common bacterial pathogen causing neonatal sepsis is:
   A. Group B streptococcus (*Streptococcus agalactiae*)
   B. *Staphylococcus aureus*
   C. *Listeria monocytogenes*
   D. *Neisseria meningitidis*
   E. *Haemophilus influenzae* type B

COMMENT

Neonatal sepsis • Newborns reveal little through history and physical examination and present with very nonspecific symptoms for a wide differential of illnesses. Therefore an infant with even minimal symptoms, such as requiring a warmer ambient environment to maintain normal body temperature, must be carefully examined with a lowered threshold for additional laboratory tests and treatment. Symptoms of neonatal sepsis can range from fever or temperature instability, hypothermia, respiratory distress, lethargy, hypotonia, apnea, seizures, feeding intolerance, abdominal distention, poor perfusion, shock, rash, unexplained jaundice, hypoglycemia, hyperglycemia, and more. There are few symptoms not associated with neonatal sepsis—erythema toxicum, a benign rash of the neonatal period, being one of them.

Risk factors • There are numerous factors that place the infant at increased risk for sepsis. Maternal factors include prolonged rupture of membranes, chorioamnionitis, maternal fever, maternal leukocytosis, uterine tenderness, and maternal genital infections or colonization such as group B streptococcus or herpes virus. Risk factors specific to the infant include low birth weight, prematurity, and male gender (the weaker sex where newborns are concerned!). Rare conditions that increase the risk of infection include congenital immune defects, galactosemia, and congenital anomalies with a skin defect such as an omphalocele or myelomeningocele.

Diagnosis • Laboratory testing for neonatal sepsis includes a complete blood count as well as cultures from blood, urine, and spinal fluid, ideally before antibiotics are instituted. Interpretation of culture results must take into account antibiotic administration to the mother immediately before delivery. A lumbar puncture should be performed in any infant suspected to have sepsis, as not all infants with meningitis have classic signs and infants with meningitis can have negative blood cultures. Urine culture, usually useful only after the first 72 hours of life, must be obtained under sterile conditions as with suprapubic aspiration or catheterization. Sepsis can result in either leukocytosis or neutropenia as well as an altered ratio of immature to total neutrophils. Chest radiographs are usually obtained to evaluate for pneumonia.

Pathogens • The most common pathogen in neonatal sepsis is group B streptococcus (GBS), especially is there is a history of maternal vaginal colonization. When maternal colonization occurs, the risk of GBS sepsis can be decreased with the use of maternal antibiotics at least 4 hours prior to delivery. Gastrointestinal bacteria, such as *E. coli*, can cause neonatal sepsis. Other pathogens specifically affecting newborns include *Listeriae*. *Haemophilus influenzae* type B, and *Neisseria meningitidis* are not common pathogens in newborns. When sepsis is suspected, antibiotics (usually ampicillin and gentamycin) should be instituted immediately and not be delayed awaiting laboratory test results.

Answers • 1-E 2-B 3-D 4-A

CASE PRESENTATION

A 9-year-old girl presents with a 12-day history of rhinorrhea and cough. The cough is worse at night. She has had occasional headaches and is now complaining of her teeth hurting. Physical exam reveals a slightly tired-appearing girl with a temperature of 101 degrees orally. She has mild tenderness to percussion over the maxillary region bilaterally. She has copious, thick rhinorrhea. Your diagnosis is acute bacterial sinusitis.

1. Which of the following organisms is the least common cause of uncomplicated acute bacterial sinusitis?
   A. *Streptoccoccus pneumoniae*
   B. *Pseudomonas aeruginosa*
   C. *Haemophilus influenzae* (non-typable)
   D. *Moraxella catarrhalis*

2. What is the mechanism of antibiotic resistance in resistant *Streptococcus pneumoniae*?
   A. Beta lactamase enzyme production
   B. Intracellular pump that excretes antibiotics
   C. Penicillin-binding protein alteration
   D. Mutations in intracellular enzymes necessary for penicillin's antimicrobial activity
   E. Blockage of cellular uptake of the antibiotic

3. What is the mechanism of antibiotic resistance in resistant *Moraxella catarrhalis*?
   A. Beta lactamase enzyme production
   B. Intracellular pump excretion of antibiotics
   C. Penicillin-binding protein alteration
   D. Mutations in intracellular enzymes necessary for penicillin's antimicrobial activity
   E. Blockage of cellular uptake of the antibiotic

4. Use of a limited computed tomography scan in sinusitis:
   A. Improves cost-effective use of antibiotics in the treatment of sinusitis
   B. Distinguishes viral and bacterial sinusitis
   C. Is unnecessary to make the diagnosis of sinusitis
   D. Is indicated in every case of sinusitis
   E. Is indicated in cases with severe symptoms

COMMENT

Sinusitis • Sinusitis is increasingly recognized as a common problem in children. Pathogens include both viruses and bacteria. The bacterial organisms that cause infection are the same organisms involved in otitis media, *Streptococcus pneumoniae*, *Moraxella catarrhalis*, and *Haemophilus influenzae*. The location of sinusitis in children depends on age as the sinuses gradually develop and enlarge. Only the maxillary and ethmoid sinuses are present at birth. The sphenoid sinus develops beginning at age 2 years and the frontal sinuses, at age 4 years. Any obstruction of sinus drainage and aeration can lead to chronic sinusitis. Causes of obstruction may include allergic rhinitis, nasal polyps, or deviated nasal septum. The major complications of bacterial sinusitis include local spread with resultant intracranial abscess formation or orbital infection and sagittal sinus thrombosis.

Diagnosis • Accurate diagnosis of this disorder can be based solely on clinical findings. Symptoms suggestive of sinusitis include cough that is usually worse at night when supine, malodorous breath, facial pain, localized headache, or tooth pain. Findings on physical examination include tenderness to percussion over the sinus and decreased transillumination of the sinus. Persistence of symptoms for greater than 10 days suggests acute bacterial sinusitis rather than viral upper respiratory infection. There has been controversy surrounding the usage of plain radiographs and computed tomography (CT) scans in the diagnosis of sinusitis. In cases that have not responded to treatment, a limited CT scan may be useful to demonstrate anatomic abnormalities or diagnose abscess formation; however, neither is necessary to make the diagnosis of sinusitis. Neither can distinguish viral infections from bacterial sinusitis.

Bacterial resistance • Antibiotic resistance in *Streptococcus pneumoniae* is due to alteration of the penicillin binding proteins. The majority of strains of *Moraxella catarrhalis* are beta lactamase producers. An increasing number of strains of *Haemophilus influenzae* are also beta lactamase producers. High-dose amoxicillin can be used in cases of resistant *Streptococcus pneumoniae* to overcome the resistance of the penicillin binding proteins. Clavulanic acid can be added to amoxicillin to inhibit the beta lactamase enzyme.

Answers • 1-B 2-C 3-A 4-C

18 SCHOOL FAILURE IN AN ADOLESCENT

● CASE PRESENTATION

A 16-year-old boy is brought by his mother with a complaint of a decline in school performance. He is in the tenth grade and has always been an honor roll student until the end of last school year, when he had difficulty in some classes but ended the year with Bs or Cs in all subjects. However, this year he is failing all subjects except band. His teachers report that he does not pay attention in class, frequently misses homework assignments, leaves completed assignments at home, and sleeps in class especially after lunch. He participated on the basketball team last year but did not try out for the team this year because he feels fatigued with exercise. At home his parents have noticed that he forgets chores, often appears to not listen, and is more argumentative. He spends more time alone in his room sleeping and appears tired. On physical examination he is sleeping on the examination table and appears tired when awoken for the examination. His weight and height have not changed since his sports preparticipation examination last spring and are appropriate for his age. His physical examination is normal.

1. Which of the conditions listed below is not typically associated with a decline in school performance?
   A. Depression
   B. Attention deficit disorder
   C. Learning disability
   D. Anorexia nervosa
   E. Substance abuse

Additional confidential history reveals that he spends most of his afternoons and weekends with several neighborhood boys but is not engaging in any organized activity. He denies depressed mood or anhedonia but does endorse increased sleeping and difficulty awakening in the morning. He has smoked cigarettes since he was 11 years old and now smokes a pack a day. He has used alcohol in the past, with his first experimentation at 12 years of age, and has used marijuana, with first use at 15 years of age. He now drinks alcohol, including beer and vodka, every weekend with his friends, usually drinking about 6 to 10 beers a night. In the last several months he has also started drinking when alone in his room or during lunch at school. He has had several episodes where he does not remember what happened after becoming drunk and stopped drinking for several weeks afterward but then resumed drinking, increasing to the current amount.

2. Which diagnostic criteria is a characteristic of substance dependence but not of substance abuse?
   A. Decline in school performance
   B. Need for increasing amounts in order to become intoxicated
   C. Continued use despite negative consequences
   D. Use over a 12-month period
   E. Majority of activities and peers focus on use

3. Which statement about adolescent substance use and abuse is not true?
   A. Alcohol is the most commonly used and abused substance
   B. Marijuana is the most commonly used and abused illegal substance
   C. Substance abuse is highest in minority adolescents from low-income families
   D. Adolescent substance abuse has increased in the last decade
   E. Physicians should include substance use screening yearly in the well-child examination of adolescent patients

4. The characteristic most indicative of substance abuse in adolescents is:
   A. Decline in school performance
   B. Dropping out of organized activities such as sports teams
   C. Increased sleeping and fatigue
   D. Change in physical appearance
   E. Peers who abuse alcohol or other drugs

● COMMENT

School failure • This is a common presenting symptom with a wide differential diagnosis in adolescent patients. Causes may include previously undetected or compensated learning disabilities or attention deficit hyperactivity disorder, psychiatric or psychological problems such as depression or anxiety, chronic illnesses, and substance use or abuse. In addition, a patient frequently has more than one of these diagnoses as several are comorbid conditions. For example, children with chronic illnesses have a higher incidence of depression. Those with attention deficit hyperactivity disorder have a greater risk of substance use or abuse, depression, and an additional learning disability. Therefore a careful history about school with vigilance for a change in performance should be a part of each adolescent medical encounter but is only a "red flag" that something is wrong, with further evaluation necessary for a specific diagnosis.

Substance use and abuse • These are two separate diagnoses, an important distinction when the physician must decide whether to reveal a history obtained from the patient in confidence. Substance experimentation is a very common adolescent experience, with up to 90% of high school seniors having had at least one drink of beer. Even frequent use is not uncommon in adolescents and may not require more intervention than confidential counseling and follow-up by the physician. However, patients with significant drug or alcohol use must be evaluated with a detailed, structured interview to determine if the criteria for substance abuse or dependence are present. Adolescents with substance abuse or dependence should be referred for treatment and their parents must be informed of the diagnosis so they can assure compliance with treatment. See Tables 1A and 1B for the diagnostic criteria of abuse and dependence.

Adolescent substance abuse has been increasing since the 1980s, with alcohol remaining the most frequently abused substance. Although some intensive skills-based interventions have had a demonstrated impact, many school-based intervention programs, such as the DARE program, have had disappointing results and have not been effective in preventing substance use and abuse. Adolescents at particular risk of substance abuse include those with a family history of substance abuse, those who have comorbid conditions such as depression or attention deficit hyperactivity disorder, adolescents from affluent families, or those who are disenfranchised from school or organized activities. An indicator of the degree of use for a patient can be a careful history of their activities and peer substance use, as adolescents do what their close friends do and will often confess to the use of others before revealing details of their own use. Of the many features suggestive of substance use, such as a decline in school performance or a change in activities, substance abuse by close friends is by far the most suggestive symptom of abuse in an adolescent patient.

Answers • 1-D 2-B 3-C 4-E

TABLE 1A • Diagnostic Criteria for Substance Abuse

A. Maladaptive pattern of substance use leading to significant impairment, as manifested by one or more of the following, occurring within a 12-month period:
  1. Substance use resulting in failure to fulfill obligations at work, school, or home
  2. Recurrent use in hazardous situations
  3. Recurrent legal problems related to substance use
  4. Continued use despite persistent or recurrent social or interpersonal problems
B. Symptoms do not meet the criteria for dependence

Adapted from the *Diagnostic and Statistical Manual of Mental Disorders IV*, 4th ed. 1994.

TABLE 1B • Diagnostic Criteria for Substance Dependence

Maladaptive pattern of substance use leading to significant impairment, as manifested by three or more of the following, occurring within the same 12-month period:
1. Tolerance, as defined by either of the following:
   (a) a need for markedly increased amounts of the substance to achieve intoxication or desired effect
   (b) marked diminished effect with continued use of the same amount
2. Withdrawal, as manifested by either of the following:
   (a) the characteristic withdrawal syndrome for the substance
   (b) the same (or closely related) substance is taken to relieve or avoid withdrawal symptoms
3. Substance is taken in larger amounts or over a longer period than intended
4. Persistent desire or unsuccessful efforts to cut down or control use
5. A great deal of time is spent in activities necessary to obtain or use the substance
6. Important social, occupational, or recreational activities are given up or reduced because of substance use
7. Use is continued despite knowledge of persistent or recurrent problems caused by use

Adapted from the *Diagnostic and Statistical Manual of Mental Disorders IV*, 4th ed. 1994.

SCROTAL PAIN IN A PREPUBERTAL BOY

● CASE PRESENTATION

A 10-year-old boy presents to the emergency department with a chief complaint of severe scrotal pain. He was asymptomatic until one hour ago when he was awoken from sleep by pain that has increased in severity since then. The pain is increased with walking and is not relieved in any position he has tried. He also complains of nausea and has vomited once. There is no history of trauma. He is not sexually active. On physical exam he is in acute distress.

1. What is the most emergent etiology of scrotal pain?
    A. Testicular torsion
    B. Hydrocele
    C. Testicular appendiceal torsion
    D. Varicocele
    E. Spermatocele

2. What physical finding is likely is this patient?
    A. Low-lying testicle
    B. Inguinal adenopathy
    C. Absent cremasteric reflex
    D. Blue dot sign
    E. Urethral discharge

3. What is the complication of delayed treatment with this diagnosis?
    A. Kawasaki disease
    B. Urinary tract infection
    C. Necrotic testis
    D. Hydrocele
    E. Henoch-Schönlein purpura

● COMMENT

Testicular torsion • Acute scrotal pain must be immediately evaluated as the differential diagnosis includes testicular torsion, a true medical emergency with a risk of necrosis of the testis and impaired fertility if the torsion is not reduced in a timely manner. Testicular torsion is the most common cause of severe acute scrotal pain and swelling in children. Although a complete exam is often difficult in patients with severe pain, physical findings may include a unilateral swollen, tender and erythematous scrotum with the affected testicle in a horizontal, superior position compared to the unaffected testicle, and absent cremasteric reflex (reflex upward retraction of the testicle). Diagnosis can be confirmed with Doppler ultrasound or testicular scan to document compromised blood flow to the testicle. Torsion can result in necrosis of the testicle and resultant impaired fertility especially if detorsion is delayed beyond six hours. Torsion of the spermatic cord is often associated with the "bell clapper" deformity, an elevated attachment of the tunica vaginalis, allowing rotation of the testis.

Torsion of the testicular appendages • Present in a similar manner as torsion of the spermatic cord (testicular torsion). As testicular appendiceal torsion causes necrosis of only the appendix of the testis and does not impact future fertility, surgical repair is not necessary. The distinctive physical finding in torsion of the testicular appendage is the "blue dot" sign, a spot of blue above the testis that is caused by the necrotic testicular appendix.

Differential diagnosis • Of scrotal pain, includes epididymitis (especially in sexually active adolescents and associated with urethral discharge), trauma, orchitis, and incarcerated hernias. Hydroceles, varicoceles, and spermatoceles also result in scrotal swelling but are usually painless.

Answers • 1-A 2-C 3-C

CASE PRESENTATION

A 3-month-old boy presents with cyanosis, irritability, and prolonged crying. His parents indicate that they were told that the patient had a murmur at his 2-month well-child examination that was thought to be an innocent flow murmur. The patient's symptoms seem to be relieved when his knees are bent up toward his chest. A chest radiograph is obtained and reveals a "boot shaped" heart.

1. What cardiac abnormalities are associated with this disorder?
   A. Ventricular septal defect, pulmonary stenosis, overriding aorta, and right ventricular hypertrophy
   B. Atrial septal defect, pulmonary stenosis, overriding aorta, and right ventricular hypertrophy
   C. Transposition of the aorta and pulmonary artery
   D. Coarctation of the aorta
   E. Tricuspid atresia

2. What electrolyte abnormality may be seen in association with this disorder?
   A. Hyponatremia
   B. Hypokalemia
   C. Hyperlipidemia
   D. Hypocalcemia
   E. Hypernatremia

3. Cyanosis in this case is due to:
   A. Left to right shunting of blood
   B. Right to left shunting of blood
   C. Hypotension
   D. Methemoglobinemia
   E. Increased pulmonary blood flow

COMMENT

Cyanotic congenital heart disease • Results from lesions that decrease pulmonary blood flow or have normal pulmonary blood flow. Conditions that decrease pulmonary blood flow include tetralogy of Fallot, pulmonary atresia and tricuspid atresia. Cyanotic conditions that have normal pulmonary blood flow have an abnormal connection between the venous and arterial systems such that the blood cannot be oxygenated. These include transposition of the great vessels, single ventricle, truncus arteriosus, and total anomalous pulmonary venous return.

Tetralogy of Fallot • The four basic characteristics of the congenital heart disease described by Fallot include a ventricular septal defect, pulmonary stenosis, an overriding aorta, and right ventricular hypertrophy. Chest radiograph reveals the classic "boot shaped heart" (also known as "coeur en sabot") due to right ventricular hypertrophy combined with the pulmonary artery abnormalities. Severity of illness depends on the degree of right ventricular outflow tract obstruction. Tetralogy of Fallot is often an isolated congenital defect, occurring equally in girls and boys and accounting for 10% of congenital heart disease. It may also be found with other anomalies as in Down syndrome or DiGeorge syndrome, with associated thymic and parathyroid hypoplasia with resultant T-cell abnormalities and hypocalcemia. Many other congenital anomalies that are not part of a syndrome complex or diagnosis are also associated with tetralogy of Fallot, such as skeletal abnormalities or hypospadias.

"Tet spells" • Increased pulmonary vascular resistance or decreased systemic vascular resistance may cause increased right to left shunting and therefore cyanosis in patients with Tetralogy of Fallot. This situation, known as a "tet spell," can result in acute distress and cyanosis. Other symptoms of a tet spell include hyperpnea, irritability, prolonged cry, and decreased intensity of the cardiac murmur. Older children often squat down when they are having a spell. Treatment of these spells is aimed at reducing the shunting. The knees-to-chest position is calming to the child and increases systemic vascular resistance. Phenylephrine increases the systemic vascular resistance. Oxygen may be used, although it is of limited value since the main problem is right to left shunting past normal lungs. Morphine may be helpful in this situation. Severe spells may result in syncope, seizures, or cardiac arrest.

Answers • 1-A 2-D 3-B

INFANT WITH WHEEZING

CASE PRESENTATION

A 4-month-old boy is brought to his physician with recurrent episodes of wheezing. The patient was first noted to wheeze at 5 weeks of age. When he had another episode of wheezing several weeks later, he was diagnosed with bronchiolitis. The test for respiratory syncytial virus at that time was negative. The wheezing improved subsequently but he has continued to wheeze intermittently since then. On physical exam, the patient is happy and active with good air movement upon auscultation. He does have a significant wheeze during expiration that is audible in all lung fields. His cardiac examination is normal. Hemoglobin oxygen saturations are normal. Upon further evaluation and after extensive testing, bronchoscopy is performed and the patient is diagnosed with tracheomalacia.

1. Initial differential diagnosis for this patient would have included:
   A. Reactive airway disease
   B. Cystic fibrosis
   C. Vascular ring or sling
   D. Gastroesophageal reflux
   E. All of the above

2. The bronchoscopy in this patient will demonstrate:
   A. Collapse of the posterior wall of the trachea toward the anterior tracheal wall
   B. Collapse of the anterior wall of the trachea toward the posterior tracheal wall
   C. Decreased fixed caliber of the lower trachea
   D. Constant bulging inward of the trachea at the level of the carina
   E. Vocal cord paralysis

3. Therapy in this child who is growing well but continues to have occasional wheezing should include:
   A. Prophylactic steroids
   B. Surgical resection of the diseased area
   C. Treatment with beta agonists
   D. Watchful waiting
   E. Thickened formula

COMMENT

Tracheomalacia • Tracheomalacia is a condition of laxity of the trachea in infants and young children, resulting from increased pliability of the cartilaginous rings. It usually resolves as the infant matures and tracheal cartilage becomes less pliable. As many patients have minimal symptoms, specific diagnostic testing is often unnecessary.

Evaluation • The differential diagnosis of an infant with wheezing is extensive and should include reactive airway disease, allergic reaction, cystic fibrosis, aspirated foreign body, gastroesophageal reflux, vascular ring or sling, cyst or polyp, and tracheoesophageal fistula. All patients with new onset of wheezing should have a chest x-ray. If any of these other illnesses are suspected by history or if a patient's symptoms are persistent and severe, further diagnostic testing may be indicated. Evaluation of the airway may include computed tomography scan, fluoroscopic evaluation or bronchoscopy. Esophagram may reveal external lesions causing tracheal compression such as vascular abnormalities. A pH probe may diagnose gastroesophageal reflux.

Prognosis • Patients will usually outgrow tracheomalacia as their tracheal cartilage matures. Therefore, watchful waiting is recommended in patients who are growing normally with no respiratory distress. Beta agonists may reduce airway stability and may worsen the symptoms. Steroids are generally not used for prophylaxis but may be used when the patient is symptomatic during an upper respiratory infection. Concurrent reflux may be treated to prevent worsening of symptoms. Surgery is reserved for severe cases.

Answers • 1-E 2-B 3-D

URINARY TRACT INFECTION

CASE PRESENTATION

A 4-month-old girl presents to the emergency department with a chief complaint of fever. On further questioning, you learn the child's fever has been as high as 102.2 degrees Fahrenheit rectally today, she has been eating less and has been fussy. Vital signs reveal temperature 102 degrees Fahrenheit, heart rate 158/minute, respiratory rate 38/minute, and blood pressure 96/68 mmHg. The patient is fussy but consolable by her mother and generally well-appearing. She is well-hydrated and well-perfused. Physical examination is normal. You decide to obtain blood and urine studies to further evaluate this patient.

1. Which of the following statements is true?
   A. Urine specimen in infants should be obtained by a clean catch specimen
   B. Urine should be sent for urinalysis alone
   C. Antibiotics should be given before urinalysis results are available as treatment should not be delayed
   D. Urinary tract infections (UTI) in infants cannot be diagnosed by history and physical
   E. UTIs in infants and young children are rarely associated with vesicoureteral reflux

2. The most common organism that causes UTI is:
   A. *Pseudomonas*
   B. *Escherichia coli*
   C. *Klebsiella*
   D. *Proteus*
   E. *Enterobacter*

3. Which antibiotic is not used in infants and young children for treatment of UTIs?
   A. Amoxicillin
   B. Aminoglycosides
   C. Sulfonamide and trimethoprim
   D. Tetracycline
   E. Macrodantin

4. What diagnostic studies are recommended to evaluate an infant or young child with a first UTI?
   A. Radiograph of kidneys, ureters, and bladder and renal ultrasound
   B. Renal ultrasound and intravenous pyelography (IVP)
   C. Renal ultrasound and voiding cystourethrography (VCUG)
   D. VCUG and IVP
   E. Renal biopsy

COMMENT

Urinary tract infections (UTI) in infants and children • As with many illnesses, infants and young children present with very nonspecific complaints when they have a UTI, often only with fever or irritability. As careful history and physical examination cannot eliminate the possibility of a UTI, infants and young children less than 2 years old who present with fever and no known source must have a urinalysis and urine culture as part of their evaluation. UTIs in children are often associated with underlying structural abnormalities or vesicoureteral reflux. Boys who are uncircumcised are more likely to have a UTI than boys who are circumcised. Risk factors for UTIs in girls include urethral irritation and contamination from bubble baths or poor hygiene, obstruction from labial adhesions, sexual activity and pregnancy. Children with underlying causes may require prophylactic antibiotics to avoid renal damage from recurrent UTIs.

Evaluation • Urine for culture must be collected under the most sterile conditions possible. Until the child has been toilet trained and a clean catch urine sample can be reliable, the sample should be obtained under sterile conditions, such as via transurethral catheterization or suprapubic bladder aspiration. Urine samples from a "bag" attached to the baby's peritoneal area are usually contaminated with multiple organisms. Antibiotics should not be given prior to obtaining cultures. As UTIs are associated with underlying abnormalities, even the first UTI in an infant, a preschool girl, or a boy at any age requires imaging of the urinary tract to evaluate for a condition that would predispose the patient to recurrent infection and the risk of renal damage. Renal ultrasonography is performed to evaluate renal and ureteral structure and dilation, and has replaced the IVP in most patients as it has less procedure-related risk. VCUG is needed to identify and grade vesicoureteral reflux. There is some controversy about when a VCUG should be obtained as studies done immediately reveal a higher rate of reflux than those done several weeks after resolution of the infection. Renal cortical scanning with DMSA may be used to assess renal scarring and to evaluate for acute pyelonephritis. Plain radiograph and renal biopsy are not routinely used to evaluate UTIs in children.

Treatment • As the most common organisms responsible for UTIs are gastrointestinal gram-negative bacteria such as *Escherichia coli*, *Klebsiella*, and *Proteus*, antibiotics used include amoxicillin and combination sulfonamide and trimethoprim. When the patient is seriously ill, intravenous aminoglycoside, often with ampicillin or another penicillin, may also be used. Tetracycline is not used in UTIs and is also not indicated for preschool children under 8 years old as it causes staining of the dental enamel. Patients should be reassessed with a repeat urine culture on antibiotics to assure sterilization of the urine. Even without any underlying condition, young children with a UTI should be followed with several urine cultures after treatment to be sure they do not have recurrent bacturia and UTIs.

Answers • 1-D 2-B 3-D 4-C

VARICELLA (CHICKEN POX)

CASE PRESENTATION

A mother brings her 12-month-old daughter to your office and is interested in giving her the varicella vaccine. She is concerned because the child spent the previous weekend with her cousins, three days ago, and now one of the cousins has vesicular lesions suspicious for "chicken pox." Neither of the cousins had received the vaccine. Your patient is currently asymptomatic.

1. Advice that you could give this parent includes:
   A. Vaccination now won't prevent illness from this exposure
   B. Vaccination now will prevent illness from this exposure
   C. The risks of vaccination outweigh the benefits
   D. 12 months is too young for varicella vaccination
   E. Vaccination now may give some protection from severe disease from this exposure and has little risk

2. Which of the following statements about the varicella vaccine is not correct?
   A. The varicella vaccine is a live virus
   B. Immunocompromised children should receive the vaccine
   C. Varicella vaccine can be given at the same time as other childhood immunizations
   D. Children older than 13 years of age require two doses of varicella vaccine
   E. The majority of adults without a reliable history of varicella are immune

3. Which clinical characteristic is not typical of varicella?
   A. Fever
   B. Malaise
   C. Generalized vesicular rash
   D. Contagious period preceding illness
   E. Anemia

4. Which statement about varicella is not true?
   A. Immunocompromised patients exposed to varicella should receive varicella-zoster immunoglobulin (VZIG) within four days.
   B. Varicella infection can cause a transient cerebellar ataxia
   C. Immunocompromised children have more severe disease
   D. Children with varicella have a higher rate of complications than do adults
   E. Intrauterine varicella infection can result in congenital birth defects

5. Which is the less likely complication of varicella infection?
   A. Bacterial cellulitis
   B. Pneumonia
   C. Dehydration
   D. Pancreatitis
   E. Hepatitis

6. What treatment is indicated for newborn infants whose mother developed varicella within five days prior to delivery or up to two days after delivery?
   A. Varicella vaccination with repeat dose one month later
   B. Isolation from the mother
   C. Bottle feeding rather than breast feeding
   D. VZIG (125 units) intramuscularly
   E. Careful follow-up and immediate varicella-zoster immune globulin if symptoms develop

COMMENT

Varicella • Varicella-zoster virus, a human herpes virus, causes a primary infection known to parents as "chicken pox." It is a highly contagious illness, spread by direct contact, droplet, or aerosol exposure from both the vesicular fluid of skin lesions and by secretions from the respiratory tract. In fact, the period during which a child is contagious begins a day or two before he or she becomes ill, making isolation difficult. The incubation period ranges from 10 to 21 days, and up to 28 days in patients who have received immunoglobulin, with an average of about two weeks, and patients are contagious until all lesions are crusted over. Symptoms include fever and malaise followed by eruptions of vesicles, described as "a dew drop on a rose petal" for their clear vesicle surrounded by erythema. While usually a relatively benign illness, albeit with great discomfort, varicella can rarely cause more serious complications such as pneumonia, hepatitis, and cerebellar ataxia, especially in immunocompromised or adult patients.

Vaccination • The varicella vaccine is recommended as part of the routine vaccination schedule, with a single dose given as early as 12 months of age. If given after 13 years of age, two doses at least one month apart are recommended. In adolescents and adults, existing immunity can be established with a reliable history of varicella infection. As varicella has been such a common illness, even most adults who do not recall previous infection are seropositive when tested. Therefore, it may be more cost-beneficial to do serologic testing on adults to determine immunity prior to giving immunizations. The vaccine is a live, attenuated virus and therefore it should not be used in some immunocompromised patients. Rare adverse events associated with immunization include localized rash, generalized varicella-like rash, and fever. While there is limited data, postexposure immunization is thought to be approximately 90% effective if given within three days of the exposure and to have no increased risk to the patient.

Treatment • Immunocompromised patients and patients at risk for severe illness, such as nonimmune pregnant women, neonates born to nonimmune mothers, and hospitalized premature infants, should receive VZIG by intramuscular injection within 96 hours of exposure to confer passive immunity and prevent or lessen their illness. Infants born to mothers who develop varicella in the perinatal period (five days before or two days after delivery) should receive VZIG (125 units intramuscularly) as soon as possible. Oral acyclovir, given immediately after onset of symptoms, may decrease the severity of illness and should be considered in adolescents and adults. Treatment in otherwise healthy children is largely symptomatic, assuring adequate hydration and limiting secondary bacterial infection of vesicular lesions.

Answers • 1-E 2-B 3-E 4-D 5-D 6-D

CASE PRESENTATION

A 10-year-old boy presents for an initial physical examination with no acute complaints. He has a past history of recurrent ear infections in infancy and his mother thinks that he may have "allergies" as he often has clear rhinorrhea, especially in the spring and fall. Family history is significant for atopic disease (asthma and allergic rhinitis). On physical examination his height is 128 cm (5%), weight is 22 kg (<5%) with no prior growth chart available. Vital signs are normal. Physical examination is significant for mouth-breathing and enlarged tonsils that are almost touching each other in his posterior pharynx.

1. Which condition is not associated with adenoidal hypertrophy?
   A. Chronic, recurrent otitis media
   B. Chronic middle ear effusion
   C. Obstructive sleep apnea
   D. Recurrent pneumonia
   E. Narrow, high palate

2. What should be the next step in evaluation of this patient?
   A. Tympanometry
   B. Anterior and lateral neck x-ray
   C. Audiometry
   D. Additional history about sleep patterns
   E. Computed tomography scan of sinuses

Further evaluation reveals that he snores loudly at night and has multiple short episodes where he does not snore followed by loud resumption of breathing. Previous measurements are obtained and reveal that he has gradually decreased in his growth velocity over the last several years, crossing from the 10–25% in height and weight to his present measurement. Sleep study confirms that he has significant obstructive sleep apnea.

3. Which condition is not associated with obstructive sleep apnea in children?
   A. Adenoidal hypertrophy
   B. Obesity
   C. Pierre Robin syndrome
   D. Down syndrome
   E. Hyperthyroidism

4. Obstructive sleep apnea can result in:
   A. Pulmonary hypertension
   B. Recurrent pneumonia
   C. Recurrent sinusitis
   D. Gastroesophageal reflux
   E. Anemia

COMMENT

Adenoidal hypertrophy • This, or enlargement of the pharyngeal tonsils and "adenoids," is common in young children but may occasionally become significant, resulting in obstruction of the upper airway and eustachian tubes. These children can have recurrent middle ear effusion and infection, chronic mouth breathing resulting in a high, narrow palate, or obstructive sleep apnea. Although surgical removal of the tonsils is performed much more circumspectly than several decades ago when it was thought to prevent streptococcal pharyngitis, it is still indicated if there is significant illness or symptoms as a result of the tonsillar enlargement.

Obstructive sleep apnea • This can usually be diagnosed with a thorough history, as the child snores so loudly that his or her entire family can describe the sleep pattern. The diagnosis is confirmed with a sleep study to measure oxygen saturation and respiratory effort during sleep. Several effects can be seen with severe sleep apnea, including growth retardation, chronic hypoxemia, and hypercapnia resulting in polycythemia, respiratory acidosis with a compensatory metabolic acidosis, and right ventricular hypertrophy leading ultimately to cor pulmonale. In addition to adenoidal hypertrophy, causes of obstructive sleep apnea include obesity (the "Pickwickian syndrome" named after an obese character in Dickens' novel, *Pickwick Papers*), Down syndrome with a large tongue and small, hypotonic pharynx, and Pierre Robin syndrome with micrognathia.

Answers • 1-D 2-D 3-E 4-A

CASE PRESENTATION

A mother presents to the emergency department stating that her 20-month-old son may have eaten 10 adult-strength acetaminophen tablets. On further questioning, you learn the tablets were 500 mg immediate-release tablets. The mother found her son playing with an empty medicine bottle and she is sure it had contained between 8 and 12 acetaminophen tablets. She had just used the bottle to take a dose of acetaminophen herself about two hours ago so she thinks the ingestion must have occurred sometime in the last two hours. The child is well-appearing and playful. He weighs 22 kg. Vital signs and physical exam are normal.

1. After your history and physical, what should the initial management of this patient include?
   A. Gastric lavage
   B. Ipecac syrup to induce vomiting
   C. Activated charcoal
   D. Serum acetaminophen level
   E. N-acetylcysteine

2. The major complication of acetaminophen toxicity is:
   A. Renal failure
   B. Hepatic damage
   C. Hearing impairment
   D. Respiratory distress
   E. Stevens-Johnson syndrome

3. Which is not indicated in regard to N-acetylcysteine therapy?
   A. Therapy should be based on the result of the four-hour serum acetaminophen level
   B. The initial dose of N-acetylcysteine is usually 140 mg/kg
   C. Subsequent doses of N-acetylcysteine are given every hour
   D. A total of 17 doses of N-acetylcysteine are given
   E. N-acetylcysteine is almost always given orally

COMMENT

Ingestion • Ingestion in pediatric patients is usually unintentional (a toddler) or intentional (an adolescent with a suicide attempt). Initial management of ingestion depends on the substance, timing, and symptoms. Induced vomiting or gastric lavage should be avoided for some substances, such as hydrocarbons, as aspiration could result in pulmonary damage. As the stomach usually empties within an hour, gastric emptying using induced vomited or lavage is of little benefit when the treatment is initiated several hours after the ingestion. Activated charcoal is beneficial for most acetaminophen ingestions, especially those that present between two and four hours after the ingestion.

Acetaminophen • This is the most commonly used antipyretic and analgesic medication in children, especially as salicylates (aspirin) are now rarely used because of their association with Reye syndrome. The toxicity of acetaminophen is caused by metabolites that at high levels overwhelm the liver's mechanism of neutralization using glutathione, resulting in hepatocellular injury. Early treatment is essential but is often difficult as there are few specific symptoms of ingestion. Therefore, initial treatment is usually based upon history and suspicion of ingestion with an acetaminophen level obtained at least four hours after ingestion guiding further treatment. The specific antidote for acetaminophen ingestion is N-acetylcysteine, which replenishes the glutathione stores in the liver. Use of N-acetylcysteine should be based upon the acetaminophen level, determining the likelihood of hepatotoxicity. The loading dose is 140 mg/kg given orally, with a 40% dose increase if activated charcoal has been given within the previous two hours as it causes some inactivation, followed by 70 mg/kg given every four hours for a total of 17 doses. The major complication of acetaminophen overdose is hepatic damage, occurring 72 to 96 hours after the initial ingestion. Adolescents are more likely to suffer liver damage than younger children and are more likely to have a level in the toxic range as their ingestions are usually intentional. Most patients recover with supportive care and have no residual damage, although severe liver damage may require liver transplantation.

Answers • 1-C 2-B 3-C

CASE PRESENTATION

A 9-year-old boy is sent for evaluation upon the recommendation of his teacher with the chief complaint of school failure. He did fairly well in school, with a B average until this year in fourth grade, which he is failing. The patient has brought a written note from his teacher that reports he often speaks out in class and is disruptive, he distracts and touches the other children, he often does not bring in his homework assignments, and while he can read he has difficulty remembering the content of his reading. Upon further history his mother confirms that he has always been very active and restless, he has difficulty completing chores he is asked to do and often appears to not be listening when she speaks to him. Physical examination is normal with appropriate height and weight.

1. Which condition is least likely as a cause of school failure in this patient?
    A. Fetal alcohol syndrome
    B. Allergic rhinitis
    C. Learning disability
    D. Hypothyroidism
    E. Hearing loss

2. The next step in the evaluation of this patient should be:
    A. Stimulant medication trial
    B. Obtain additional objective information from parents and teachers
    C. Thyroid function tests
    D. Antihistamine medication trial
    E. Referral for counseling

Further evaluation reveals elevated hyperactivity and inattention on psychological instruments completed by the parents and teacher consistent with attention deficit hyperactivity disorder (ADHD), and normal hearing and vision screening tests. The patient is started on a trial of stimulant medication with an excellent response, with less physically hyperactive and impulsive behavior in class; however, he continues to have difficulty with reading comprehension.

3. What is the most likely cause of this patient's difficulty with reading?
    A. Mental retardation
    B. Tourette syndrome
    C. Learning disability in reading
    D. Inadequate dose of stimulant medication
    E. Incorrect diagnosis of ADHD

COMMENT

School failure • This is a nonspecific presenting symptom with a wide differential diagnosis depending on the age of the child. In elementary school-age children a change in school performance may be the subtle presentation of an unrecognized underlying illness or exposure to abuse or neglect. Several chronic illnesses make children fidgety, such as allergic rhinitis (hypothyroidism should make a child less active and have growth failure). Medications, such as albuterol, can affect behavior and concentration. Problems such as hearing loss or poor vision should always be considered. Inattention and hyperactivity may be a consequence of prenatal exposure to alcohol, cocaine, or nicotine or a result of lead poisoning. However with the changing demands at each grade level, school failure, especially beginning at fourth grade, is often due to a learning disability, ADHD, or both.

Attention deficit hyperactivity disorder • This is a clinically diagnosed condition comprised of features of inattention alone (ADD) or inattention combined with hyperactivity (ADHD) that have been present since early childhood, are seen in at least two settings (home and school), and are severe enough to cause an impairment. The diagnosis cannot be made solely upon observation of the child during a physical examination but must be substantiated with information from both parents and teachers, ideally as a well validated psychological instrument that has been normalized for children at the same age. ADD/ADHD often may be an inherited condition, usually as an autosomal dominant trait with variable expression. In several research studies patients have been found to have a defect involving the dopamine system located in the area of the brain that controls alertness and attention with a specific gene involving either the dopamine receptor or transporter identified in several families. Another inherited condition, Tourette syndrome, may include the symptoms of ADHD with other symptoms such as tics and occasionally coprolalia.

Comorbid conditions • Comorbid conditions are present in many patients with ADD/ADHD and must always be considered, especially if school difficulty continues after treatment of the symptoms of ADD/ADHD. Many patients with ADD/ADHD also have a learning disability, a significant discrepancy between abilities in a child with normal intelligence, often in reading. Other comorbid conditions that must be considered, especially as the patient becomes an adolescent, are oppositional defiant disorder, conduct disorder, depression, and substance use or abuse. Children with ADD/ADHD have a higher rate of injury and motor vehicle accidents and should have particularly vigilant injury prevention counseling throughout childhood.

Answers • 1-D 2-B 3-C

CASE PRESENTATION

An 8-year-old boy presents with a chief complaint of runny nose for the last several weeks. On further questioning, you learn that symptoms of sneezing, rhinorrhea, nasal congestion, and itching eyes have been present intermittently for about two years and have gradually worsened. It is unclear if the symptoms are seasonal or after exposure to specific environmental allergens. The patient lives in a home with parents who both smoke, a dog, and a cat. On physical examination he is appropriate weight and height with dark circles under his eyes, upturned nose, slightly injected conjunctiva, clear bilateral nasal discharge with pale, boggy nasal mucosa, and no tenderness to percussion of his sinuses. The rest of his physical examination is normal.

1. Which clinical sign is not associated with allergic rhinitis?
    A. Boggy nasal mucosa
    B. Allergic salute
    C. Transverse nasal crease
    D. Allergic shiners with Dennie lines
    E. Fever

2. Which of the following allergic diseases is most frequently seen in patients who also have allergic rhinitis?
    A. Urticaria
    B. Eczema
    C. Food allergies
    D. Anaphylaxis
    E. Drug allergies

3. Which treatment is not indicated for allergic rhinitis?
    A. Avoidance of environmental triggers
    B. Antihistamines
    C. Topical corticosteroids
    D. Prophylactic antibiotics
    E. Immunotherapy

COMMENT

Allergic rhinitis • This is a very common illness, affecting approximately 5 to 9% of children, with increasing prevalence in older children. Exposures that cause symptoms vary for individual patients but may include seasonal environmental allergens such as pollens of trees, grasses, and weeds, indoor environmental allergens such as dust mites, feathers, mold, and pet dander (most commonly cats), and passive tobacco exposure. Patients with allergic rhinitis commonly have chronic, recurrent symptoms of sneezing, clear rhinorrhea, nasal congestion, pruritus of nose and eyes, conjunctivitis, and cough.

Diagnosis • Physical findings that differentiate allergic rhinitis from an upper respiratory tract infection include boggy, pale nasal mucosa caused by the mucus membrane edema rather than swollen, erythematous nasal mucosa and a nasal discharge that is usually clear. Children can have dark circles under their eyes referred to as allergic shiners, often also with an extra crease in their lower eyelid (Dennie line). Recurrent rhinnorrhea causes a child to push up on the tip of his or her nose (the allergic salute) resulting in a transverse nasal crease at the end of the nose. Patients often are chronic mouth breathers and may have unrecognized obstructive sleep apnea. Although children with allergic rhinitis are at risk of developing infection in the obstructed spaces of the face (otitis media and sinusitis) resulting in acute illness, fever itself is not a clinical sign of allergic rhinitis alone. Other forms of atopic disease are often seen in patients with allergic rhinitis, the most common of which are eczema and asthma. Often there is a family history of atopic illness.

Treatment • The most important aspect of treatment is avoidance of exposure to specific allergens that trigger symptoms in an individual patient, often a difficult task. Environmental changes should be instituted for every patient, with time devoted by the physician to discussion of suggested changes. Symptomatic treatment and prevention of illness usually includes antihistamines, especially the nonsedating, extended release products. If nasal congestion is significant, temporary symptomatic relief may also include sympathomimetic decongestant. Patients with chronic, recurrent symptoms benefit from local use of corticosteroids or cromolyn in the form of nasal sprays. Immunotherapy, designed to include the specific allergens of an individual patient and given as repeated injection, can be very useful when these other treatment options are inadequate to control recurrent symptoms and when skin testing is positive for specific allergens that correlate with symptoms.

Answers • 1-E 2-B 3-D

CASE PRESENTATION

An 18-month-old boy is seen for a routine well-child examination with no complaints. His family history is negative. His immunizations are up to date. He has had normal development and is now able to walk, stoop down and recover, feed himself, and say "mama" and "dada." He eats table food but also still takes bottles with whole milk. Physical examination is normal with a weight of 15 kg (>95%). Laboratory testing reveals the results below:

Hemoglobin	10.0 g/dl (normal 10.5 to 14.0 for 6 months to 6 years old)
Hematocrit	33% (normal 33 to 42 for 6 months to 6 years old)
MCV	69 fl (normal 70 to 74)
RDW	15.5% (normal 11.5 to 14.5%)

1. The most likely etiology of this patient's anemia is:
   A. Lead poisoning
   B. Blood loss
   C. Iron deficiency
   D. Folate deficiency
   E. Thalassemia
2. The underlying cause in this patient is probably:
   A. Cow's milk allergy
   B. Inadequate iron intake
   C. Inadequate prenatal iron stores
   D. Malabsorption
   E. Abnormal transferrin
3. What laboratory test would confirm this diagnosis?
   A. Peripheral blood smear
   B. Hemoglobin electrophoresis
   C. Serum ferritin
   D. Erythrocyte sedimentation rate
   E. Platelet count

COMMENT

Anemia • Anemia is such a common problem in infancy that routine well-child care recommendations include screening regularly throughout early childhood and then again during adolescence. The most common form of anemia in young children is microcytic anemia, usually caused by iron deficiency, although lead toxicity can lead to identical hematologic abnormalities and must always be considered. While acute blood loss presents with normocytic anemia with a reticulocytosis, chronic blood loss depletes the body's iron stores and results in a microcytic anemia, no longer with reticulocytosis. Thalassemia is a rare hemoglobinopathy resulting in a congenital microcytic anemia with a decreased RDW. Folate deficiency is rarely seen in children and causes a macrocytic anemia.

Iron deficiency • Iron deficiency in young children is usually secondary to inadequate dietary intake. The classic presentation is the child described in this case, a plump toddler consuming a large amount of cow's milk in his bottle. Iron deficiency may also be caused by inadequate iron stores at birth such as in premature infants. Excessive iron demands as with gastrointestinal blood loss may be seen with cow's milk protein sensitivity, an intestinal polyp, or rarely a Meckel diverticulum. Although rare causes of blood loss and iron deficiency are numerous, in clinical practice if the presentation is consistent with inadequate dietary iron in a toddler, response to iron supplementation is often the only diagnostic test necessary. However, patients with severe iron deficiency may also be found to have decreased serum ferritin with a characteristic RBC appearance on peripheral smear (microcytic, hypochromic cells with poikilocytosis). Erythrocyte sedimentation rate should be normal in patients with iron deficiency due to inadequate dietary intake. Although a variety of platelet abnormalities (either thrombocytosis or thrombocytopenia) may rarely occur, they are uncommon and not specific.

Answers • 1-C 2-B 3-C

CASE PRESENTATION

A 17-year-old girl presents for a yearly well-child exam with no complaints. On review of her medical record, she has lost 20 lbs. since her visit last year. On further history, she admits to increased exercise and now runs at least five miles a day. She also has not had a menstrual cycle for the past four months, although she had menarche at age 12 and normal, monthly cycles since age 13. She feels that she is "fat" and wants to lose additional weight, limits her daily caloric intake with a very low fat diet and frequently skips meals. She denies self-induced vomiting, use of laxatives or diuretics, or binge eating. On physical examination she has a weight of 80 lbs (<5%), height 62 inches (25%), body mass index 15 (<5%) with vital signs of temperature 97.6 degrees F, heart rate 55/minute, respiratory rate 16/minute, and blood pressure 110/60 mmHg with no orthostatic changes. On physical examination she has increased lanugo hair and dry coarse skin but otherwise physical examination is normal with Tanner stage V breasts and genitalia.

1. Which characteristic is not a major diagnostic criteria for anorexia nervosa?
   A. Refusal to maintain body weight at or above minimal normal weight for age
   B. Intense fear of gaining weight or becoming fat
   C. Excessive exercise in order to lose weight
   D. Disturbance in the way body weight or shape is experienced
   E. Amenorrhea in postmenarcheal females

2. Further assessment of this patient, which should include an EKG as an important cardiac complication of anorexia nervosa, is:
   A. Tachycardia
   B. Bradycardia
   C. Prolonged QTc
   D. Hypertension with left ventricular strain
   E. Peaked p waves due to hyperkalemia

3. Which of the following is not associated with an increased risk of anorexia nervosa?
   A. Upper socioeconomic status
   B. Female gender
   C. Poor school performance
   D. Caucasian race
   E. Family history of anorexia nervosa

4. Osteoporosis in patients with anorexia nervosa is best prevented by:
   A. Increased weight-bearing exercise
   B. Estrogen therapy
   C. Decreased isometric exercise
   D. Weight gain
   E. Calcium supplementation

COMMENT

Anorexia nervosa • This affects approximately 5% of young women and dieting behaviors are becoming increasingly common in even elementary age girls. Factors that are associated with a higher incidence of anorexia nervosa include female gender, higher socioeconomic status, white race, and a family history of an eating disorder. Patients are usually excellent students, involved in many activities. Comorbid conditions that occur in these patients include depression, anxiety disorder, and obsessive-compulsive disorder.

Diagnostic criteria • The DSM IV lists four diagnostic criteria that must be met to diagnose anorexia nervosa: (1) refusal to maintain body weight at or above a minimally normal weight (less than 85% expected or failure to gain as expected in younger children), (2) intense fear of gaining weight or becoming fat even though underweight, (3) disturbance in the way one's weight and shape is experienced with undue influence on self-evaluation or denial of the seriousness of the current low body weight, and (4) amenorrhea in postmenarcheal females (this criteria need not be met in premenarcheal girls). Anorexia nervosa may present as the restricting type with limited caloric intake or the binge-eating/purging type with episodes of binge-eating, self-induced vomiting, or misuse of laxatives, diuretics, or enemas. Although patients often use excessive exercise as a type of purging behavior, it is not a separate specific diagnostic criteria.

Cardiac complications • Dysrhythmias are a cause of death in patients with anorexia nervosa, usually secondary to a conduction delay. Electrolyte abnormalities may also cause potentially fatal dysrhythmia. For this reason, an EKG with calculation of a corrected QT interval should be obtained in patients with an eating disorder and repeated periodically until they have regained significant weight. Bradycardia, and not tachycardia, is found in most patients with anorexia nervosa.

Osteoporosis • Adolescent and adult osteoporosis is a serious long-term consequence of anorexia nervosa caused by the hypoestrogenic secondary amenorrhea seen in these patients as well as their malnutrition and poor calcium intake. Although weight-bearing exercise increases bone density in normal women, in these patients exercise contributes to inadequate calories and continued weight loss such that usually exercise must be initially limited or curtailed. While estrogen replacement is often necessary in order to maximize bone calcium deposit before the end of adolescence and nutritional counseling should include adequate calcium, the primary treatment is still weight gain.

Answers • 1-C 2-C 3-C 4-D

CASE PRESENTATION

A 12-year-old boy presents for an annual well-child examination with no complaints. He has had a history of asthma since he was 4 years old with one previous hospitalization, but he states that his asthma is now well controlled. On further history he often has a nonproductive cough, especially in the spring season and also immediately after exercise. He uses an albuterol inhaler (without a spacer) several times a week when he has coughing or feels a "tightness in his chest." He is awakened with a cough, occasionally associated with wheezing, about twice a week. On physical examination he is appropriate weight and height with vital signs including a heart rate of 80/minute, respiratory rate of 20/minute, and blood pressure of 100/60 mmHg. He has clear auscultation of his chest when breathing quietly but has scattered, diffuse wheezing at the end of forced expiration. His peak flow is 70% of the predicted value.

1. Which of the following factors is not used to determine the severity of asthma?
   A. Frequency of symptoms of asthma
   B. Frequency of nocturnal symptoms of asthma
   C. Frequency of acute exacerbations
   D. Symptoms of asthma with activity
   E. Number of respiratory infections in the last year

2. Which of the following symptoms of respiratory distress is not typical of patients with asthma?
   A. Wheezing
   B. Shortened expiratory phase
   C. Accessory muscle use
   D. Dyspnea
   E. Tachypnea

3. Predicted peak expiratory flow rate is determined based on the patient's:
   A. Weight
   B. Height
   C. Chest circumference
   D. Gender
   E. Race

4. Based on the history and physical examination of this patient, the classification of his asthma severity would be:
   A. Mild with intermittent symptoms
   B. Mild with persistent symptoms
   C. Moderate with persistent symptoms
   D. Severe with persistent symptoms
   E. Status asthmaticus

COMMENT

Asthma • Asthma (reactive airway disease) is the most common chronic illness of childhood, affecting approximately 10% of children. It is an obstructive lung disease that involves hyperreactivity and inflammation of the airways and the capacity to reverse the obstructive process spontaneously or with treatment. Asthma has a genetic component and is associated with a family history of asthma or other atopic disease. It is also associated with exposure to smoking in early childhood. Although the treatment of asthma has greatly improved in the last 20 years, the overall incidence and morbidity of this illness continues to increase, especially in children living in poverty. Ongoing, preventive medical care is essential, rather than episodic treatment of acute episodes. In fact, patients with chronic, unrecognized symptoms and overuse of albuterol inhalers are those who can suddenly decompensate with status asthmaticus. A careful medical history can determine which patients have more severe disease and require additional medical intervention (see Table 2). Symptoms and tests determining the classification of asthma severity include frequency of symptoms, use of medication, and exacerbations, and tests of lung function (either forced expiratory volume in one second or peak expiratory flow rate). While respiratory illnesses may initiate an exacerbation of asthma, the frequency of respiratory illnesses is not related to asthma severity.

Physical findings consistent with respiratory distress during an acute exacerbation include tachypnea, tachycardia, use of accessory muscles for respiration, and wheezing. As asthma is an obstructive pulmonary disease, patients will have a prolonged expiratory phase of respiration. In severe status asthmaticus additional findings may include cyanosis, dyspnea, decreased air movement with a quieter exam on ascultation and an increased pulsus paradoxus >20 mmHg (the change in systolic blood pressure between inspiration and expiration). The measure of pulmonary function that is most often used in the pediatric office is the predicted peak expiratory flow rate (PEFR) that is compared to the normal mean adjusted by the height of the patient. PEFR can be used to monitor the severity of illness and response to medication for individual patients. As PEFR is not as accurate or thorough as pulmonary function testing, patients with severe disease or who do not respond as expected to therapy should be referred for additional testing.

Answers • 1-E 2-B 3-B 4-C

TABLE 2 • Classification of Asthma Severity			
Clinical Severity	Symptoms	Night-time Symptoms	Lung Function
Mild, intermittent	Symptoms ≤2 times a week Asymptomatic and normal PEFR between exacerbations Exacerbations are brief	≤2/month	FEV1 or PEFR ≥80% PEFR variability <20%
Mild, persistent	Symptoms >2 times a week but <1 a day Exacerbations may affect activity	>2/month	FEV1 or PEFR ≥80% PEFR variability 20–30%
Moderate, persistent	Daily symptoms Daily use of inhaled β agonist Exacerbations affect activity Exacerbations ≥2/week	>1/week	FEV1 or PEFR >60 but <80% PEFR variability >30%
Severe, persistent	Continual symptoms Limited exercise Frequent exacerbations	Frequent	FEV1 or PEFR ≤60% PEFR variability >30%

From the National Asthma Education and Prevention Program, National Heart, Lung, and Blood Institute Expert Panel Report 2: Guidelines for the Diagnosis and Management of Asthma, Washington DC, NIH Publication no. 97-4051, July 1997.

CASE PRESENTATION

A 12-year-old boy presents for evaluation of his growth. His parents are very concerned because he is shorter than his friends and classmates. He was a full-term, appropriate for gestational age infant, grew normally during infancy, and has continued to grow at a steady rate. He has been well, with no significant past medical history or chronic illnesses. His parents are both normal stature, at the 50th percentile. On physical exam, his weight and height are just below the fifth percentile on the male growth chart with a body mass index (BMI) at the 50th percentile for his age. The physical exam is normal with no pubic hair and genitalia, Tanner stage 1 of secondary sexual development (prepubertal). See growth chart on p. 34.

1. Of the following elements of history, the most important in determining the specific differential diagnosis in a case of short stature is:
   A. Height of the mother
   B. Height of the father
   C. Family history of short stature
   D. Pattern of growth velocity (growth curve)
   E. Family history of delayed puberty

Additional history reveals that the father was a "late bloomer," still growing for several years after he went to college. On further testing, the patient's wrist x-ray reveals a bone age that is slightly delayed at 9½ years.

2. The diagnosis of constitutional growth delay is supported by what finding?
   A. Midparental height at 50th percentile
   B. Bone age equal to height age
   C. Growth velocity greater than normal for age
   D. Normal intelligence
   E. Weight less than fifth percentile

3. You counsel this patient and his parents that:
   A. He will have a slow, steady growth velocity until reaching his final adult height at the fifth percentile
   B. He will have a gradually decreasing growth velocity and require growth hormone treatment to have a normal adult height
   C. He will have a normal increase in growth velocity with puberty and will continue growing until a later age than most boys, reaching a normal final adult height
   D. He will require caloric supplementation to assure normal growth velocity
   E. He should be tested for hypothyroidism as his bone age is delayed

COMMENT

Growth • Concerns about growth and development are the most frequent questions parents ask pediatricians. Knowledge of the normal sequence of puberty and the common conditions affecting development are essential. Fortunately, with the simple clinical tools of a detailed history and a growth chart documenting height and weight over time, a differential diagnosis can usually be identified. The change in growth velocity over time and the change in height percentile with the comparable weight chart (such as body mass index, BMI) is invaluable. Some examples of findings with specific conditions are listed in Table 3.

In evaluating a patient with short stature, it is important to determine the heights of the parents to account for genetic influence. Children usually grow to be within 10 cm (4 in.) of their midparental height. Therefore, the midparental height percentile can be assumed to be the expected height percentile for the patient. The child's expected height can be calculated based on mid-parental height as calculated below:

For boys:

$$\text{Mid-parental height} = \frac{\text{father's height} + \text{mother's height} + 13 \text{ cm}}{2}$$

For girls:

$$\text{Mid-parental height} = \frac{\text{father's height} + \text{mother's height} - 13 \text{ cm}}{2}$$

Constitutional growth delay • This is often a familial condition, usually affecting fathers and sons. Patients have normal growth parameters at birth and grow normally in early infancy followed by a very gradual deceleration in growth velocity causing them to cross percentiles on the growth chart during childhood. In childhood they continue to grow at a steady rate of about 5 cm per year or more, following the lower normal percentiles of the growth curve. In early adolescence they have delayed puberty and fall below the normal percentile as other children have a pubertal growth spurt. As bone maturation reflects androgen exposure, their bone age will be delayed and will be equivalent to the bone age that would be found in a 50th percentile child for that height (bone age = height age). Patients with constitutional growth delay ultimately begin pubertal development, rarely requiring hormonal treatment, and catch up with an increased growth velocity until a later age, attaining normal final adult stature.

Answers • 1-D 2-B 3-C

34 SHORT STATURE

2 to 20 years: Boys
Stature-for-age and Weight-for-age percentiles

NAME _____
RECORD # _____

Mother's Stature _____ Father's Stature _____

Date	Age	Weight	Stature	BMI*

*To Calculate BMI: Weight (kg) ÷ Stature (cm) ÷ Stature (cm) x 10,000
or Weight (lb) ÷ Stature (in) ÷ Stature (in) x 703

Published May 30, 2000 (modified 11/21/00).
SOURCE: Developed by the National Center for Health Statistics in collaboration with
the National Center for Chronic Disease Prevention and Health Promotion (2000).
http://www.cdc.gov/growthcharts

CDC
SAFER·HEALTHIER·PEOPLE™

TABLE 3 • Characteristics of Conditions Causing Short Stature						
Diagnosis	Growth Velocity	BMI	Puberty	Bone Age	Other Features
Acquired hypothyroidism	Severely decreased	Increased	Delayed	Very delayed	Myxedema, lethargy
Growth hormone deficiency	Decreased since birth	Normal	Variable	Delayed	Rounded facial features
Constitutional growth delay	Slightly decreased after infancy with delayed pubertal growth spurt	Normal	Delayed	Delayed, equal to height age	Positive family history
Precocious puberty	Early pubertal growth spurt and decreased final height	Normal	Early	Advanced	Advanced secondary sexual development
Skeletal dysplasia	Decreased since birth	Variable	Normal	Normal	Skeletal abnormalities, disproportionate body habitus
Chronic illness	Decreased	Decreased	Delayed	Delayed	Variable with each illness

CASE PRESENTATION

A 16-year-old girl presents with fatigue for the last two months. She has trouble awakening in the morning and has been missing school several days a week. She usually takes a nap in the afternoon and goes to sleep by 10 p.m. each evening. She feels that she has less exercise tolerance but is not involved in any sports and is not physically active so is unsure about an exact change. She is able to walk up the stairs at home and at school without dyspnea. On further questioning she reports a decreased appetite but denies vomiting or abdominal pain. Review of systems is otherwise negative with no insomnia, fever, weight loss, or amenorrhea.

She lives with both parents and a younger brother and there have been no recent changes or increased conflict at home. She is in the 10th grade and has had a slight decline in school performance, from straight As last year to As and Bs this year. Because of excessive school absences, she is failing this semester, although she maintains a B average in all subjects. She has dropped out of several school activities, including the school yearbook and track team, as she doesn't have enough energy for afterschool activities. She denies smoking, substance use, or sexual activity.

Physical examination reveals a height of 163 cm (50%), weight 75 kg (90 to 95%) (a 7 kg increase from her sports preparticipation examination six months ago), body mass index 27 (90 to 95%), heart rate 85/minute, respiratory rate 20/minute, blood pressure 110/70 mmHg. Physical examination is significant for complaints of muscle and joint tenderness diffusely with palpation but without point tenderness, joint swelling, or arthritis. Physical examination is otherwise normal.

1. Which diagnosis is least likely based on the history and physical examination for this patient?
   A. Hypothyroidism
   B. Chronic fatigue syndrome
   C. Depression
   D. Celiac disease
   E. Collagen vascular disease

2. What further evaluation would best contribute to determining the diagnosis?
   A. Complete blood count and erythrocyte sedimentation rate
   B. Additional history
   C. Antigliand antibody level
   D. Thyroid function tests
   E. Psychological testing

Upon further questioning the patient endorses several other symptoms including depressed mood every day for most of the day, anhedonia, and inability to concentrate in school. She denies feelings of worthlessness.

3. What additional evaluation or treatment must be conducted at this visit and not delayed until a return appointment?
   A. Obtain thyroid function tests
   B. Refer the patient for counseling
   C. Prescribe antidepressant medication
   D. Ascertain risk of suicide and safety at home
   E. Request homebound education from school system

COMMENT

Depression • Presents with many subtle physical complaints and only rarely with a complaint of "depressed mood." It is common among adolescents, affecting about 5% of otherwise healthy teens. The incidence of depression is higher in girls than boys, in Caucasian patients than in African-American, in patients with chronic illnesses, and in patients with a family history of depression. Primary care physicians must be skilled in diagnosing and treating depression as patients are much more likely to see their physician for the assorted somatic symptoms than they are to seek counseling. In fact, most adolescents who commit suicide have had an appointment with their primary physician within the month prior to their death but their depression often was not recognized. Although the term "depressed" is used too commonly as an adjective describing mood, depression is an illness defined by specific diagnostic criteria that are easily obtained in a thorough, confidential history (see Table 4). Adolescents may suffer from several types of depression including adjustment disorder or bereavement in addition to major depression, each of which has its own diagnostic criteria.

Evaluation • Should always include a careful history and physical examination to eliminate other illnesses, substance use or medication effects that can masquerade as depression. Usually history and examination alone are adequate, however, adolescents with depressive symptoms are often tested for hypothyroidism as the symptoms of this condition overlap those of depression and are also insidious in onset. The immediate evaluation of an adolescent with depression must include ascertainment of suicide risk, including safety in the home. The presence of a gun in the home greatly increases the chances of a completed suicide, especially with adolescent boys. Girls are more likely to attempt suicide, however, boys are more likely to commit suicide, often because they choose more lethal methods, such as firearms or hanging. Patients with a high risk of suicide (prior history of an attempt, current suicidal ideation and/or plan, and those who will not contract for safety) require emergency hospitalization.

Treatment • Treatment of adolescent depression has greatly benefited from new antidepressants, such as the selective serotonin reuptake inhibitors, as the risk of an overdose is much lower than with the tricyclic antidepressants. Adolescents with significant impairment due to depression respond to medication but usually not until about one month after starting treatment. However as adolescent depression often includes many family and individual difficulties, patients should also be referred for individual and family counseling.

Answers • 1-D 2-B 3-D

TABLE 4 • Criteria for Major Depressive Episode

A. Five or more of the following symptoms during the same two-week period, at least one of which is (1) or (2)
   (1) Depressed mood most of the day, nearly every day
   (2) Diminished interest or pleasure in almost all activities (anhedonia)
   (3) Significant weight change (>5%) or change in appetite
   (4) Insomnia or hypersomnia
   (5) Psychomotor agitation or retardation
   (6) Fatigue nearly every day
   (7) Feelings of worthlessness or excessive guilt nearly every day
   (8) Diminished ability to think or concentrate
   (9) Recurrent thoughts of death or suicide
B. Symptoms do not meet criteria for a mixed episode
C. Symptoms cause significant impairment
D. Symptoms are not due to substance or medication use or medical condition
E. Symptoms are not better accounted for by bereavement

Adapted from the *Diagnostic and Statistical Manual of Mental Disorders IV*, 4th ed. 1994.

INFANT WITH DEVELOPMENTAL DELAY

CASE PRESENTATION

A mother brings her 6-month-old child to your office with concerns about his developmental skills.

1. What developmental task would you expect this child to have achieved?
   A. Pull to stand
   B. Know one word
   C. Reach for an object
   D. Play pat-a-cake
   E. Say "mama and dada" specifically

2. Which of the following areas of development is not assessed when screening the development of infants?
   A. Gross motor skills
   B. Fine motor skills
   C. Language skills
   D. Cognitive skills
   E. Social skills

3. Which primitive reflex should have disappeared by 6 months of age?
   A. Toe grasp
   B. Moro
   C. Parachute
   D. Protective equilibrium

COMMENT

Normal infant development • The developmental skills assessed in infants are divided into four categories: gross motor, fine motor, social, and language. Standardized screening tools, such as the Denver Developmental Screening Test II, can be used to quickly evaluate developmental skills and screen for a possible delay. Cognitive abilities are impossible to assess in infants. Some tasks of normal development that should be achieved by each different age are listed in Table 5.

Primitive reflexes • There are numerous primitive reflexes in infants that are present at birth and disappear at different ages. Persistence of these primitive reflexes beyond these specific ages may indicate developmental delay. The Moro reflex, an outstretching of arms with a startle that are then brought to the center, disappears by 4 months. The hand grasp, reflexive grip around anything placed in the palm, disappears by 3 months, and the similar toe grasp, by 8–15 months. The parachute response, also referred to as lateral propping, which is the extension of a child's extremities when the child is falling in the ventral position, does not appear until 4 to 6 months. The protective equilibrium response appears at 4 to 6 months and persists voluntarily.

TABLE 5 • Normal Infant Development

Age (months)	Gross Motor	Fine Motor	Social	Language
6	Rolls over	Reaches for and grasps object	Feeds self	Imitates speech
9	Stands holding	Takes two cubes	Feeds self	Jabbers
12	Stands two seconds	Bangs cubes together	Plays pat-a-cake	Mama/dada specific

Answers • 1-C 2-D 3-B

CASE PRESENTATION

The patient is a male infant, born by vaginal delivery to a 33-year-old gravida 2 para 2 mother at 36 weeks gestation following premature labor for one week. The amniotic membranes were ruptured at delivery with a large amount of clear fluid noted. Physical examination is significant for a hypotonic infant, in no acute distress, with a protuberant tongue, flattened facial features and upward slanting palpebral fissures with epicanthal folds, and a single transverse palmar crease.

1. The most likely diagnosis for this patient is:
   A. Trisomy 13
   B. Trisomy 18
   C. Trisomy 21
   D. Meconium aspiration
   E. Congenital muscular dystrophy

The patient does well for the first several hours of life but then vomits immediately after attempting the first feeding. Physical examination at that time reveals a heart rate of 180/minute, respiratory rate of 36/minute, and a slightly full abdomen but is otherwise normal.

2. The test most likely to diagnose the cause of this patient's vomiting is:
   A. Complete blood count
   B. Blood glucose
   C. Echocardiography
   D. Abdominal x-ray
   E. Arterial blood gas

3. Which of the following medical conditions is not associated with Down syndrome?
   A. Congenial heart disease
   B. Hypothyroidism
   C. Congenital hip dislocation
   D. Leukemia
   E. Ptosis

COMMENT

Down syndrome • It is the most common chromosomal aneuploidy in live births, usually recognized immediately after delivery by the classic constellation of dysmorphic features: hypotonia, flattened facial features and occiput, upward slanted palpebral fissures with epicanthal folds, a large protuberant tongue, and small hands with a single transverse palmar crease and clinodactyly (incurved) fifth finger. Infants with Down syndrome are more likely to be born prematurely and are usually small at birth. Causes of Down syndrome include trisomy 21 (95% of patients) as well as translocation of a segment of 21, with the recurrence risk dependent on the chromosomal etiology. The risk of trisomy 21 increases with maternal age.

Congenital defects • Congenital defects in patients with Down syndrome are common, especially congenital heart disease, which may be seen in about one-third of patients, ranging from simple ventricular septal defects to more severe endocardial cushion defects. Other congenital birth defects associated with Down syndrome include congenital hip dysplasia, vertebral anomalies especially atlantoaxial instability, and intestinal atresias or obstruction as with an annular pancreas or malrotation. In this patient with prenatal polyhydramnios and vomiting with initial feeding, intestinal obstruction must be considered. X-ray will reveal a stomach full of air and a "double bubble" diagnosing this patient's duodenal atresia.

Medical conditions • Such that may develop later in infancy or childhood include recurrent, chronic otitis media (almost universally requiring myringotomy tubes), autoimmune illnesses such as hypothyroidism and diabetes mellitus, very elevated immature leukocytes (usually mimicking leukemia but also sometimes true leukemia), and strabismus. As adults, patients with Down syndrome are at risk of early onset Alzheimer dementia.

Answers • 1-C 2-D 3-E

RECURRENT WHEEZING AND PNEUMONIA

CASE PRESENTATION

A 4-year-old boy presents with cough and fever for the past day. His temperature has been as high as 103 degrees at home and he has a constant, nonproductive cough, not related to position. He is not eating as well as usual but continues to drink adequately. On physical examination his vital signs are temperature 102.5, heart rate 110/minute, respiratory rate 38/minute, and blood pressure 100/60 mmHg. He is slightly dyspneic with some accessory muscle use for respiration but no observed cyanosis. On ascultation of his chest, he has rales and wheezing in the left lower lung. Percutaneous oxygen saturation is 90% in room air.

1. What is the most likely pathogen that causes bacterial pneumonia in a preschool child?
   A. *Streptococcus pneumoniae*
   B. *Staphylococcus aureus*
   C. *Mycoplasma pneumoniae*
   D. *Haemophilus influenzae* type B
   E. Group A *Streptococcus*

Evaluation confirms a left lower lobe infiltrate on x-ray and an elevated white blood count with increased total and immature neutrophils. Blood culture is negative. The patient responds to treatment with oxygen and intravenous antibiotics followed by a course of oral antibiotics after discharge to home. On evaluation two weeks after discharge, he is afebrile and in no respiratory distress. On physical examination he has scattering wheezing in the left chest but no rales. Further history reveals that he had another episode of pneumonia, also in the left lobe, about four months ago.

2. What further diagnostic test is indicated in this patient?
   A. Sweat test
   B. Repeat x-ray with inspiratory and expiratory views
   C. Total immunoglobulin level
   D. Bone marrow aspirate
   E. Immunoglobulin A level

3. Which illness usually does not cause wheezing in children?
   A. Pneumonia
   B. Asthma
   C. Congenital heart disease
   D. Foreign body aspiration
   E. Croup

COMMENT

Foreign body aspiration • Sometimes all that wheezes is not asthma and the presenting diagnosis is not the only answer. This patient illustrates a child with seemingly straightforward bacterial pneumonia, however, further evaluation reveals an underlying cause, an aspirated foreign body. Children, especially toddlers, are notorious in their ability to insert objects into body cavities! In the lungs, peanuts cause particular problems when aspirated because of local bronchial swelling resulting in greater obstruction of the airway. Pediatricians counsel parents to avoid feeding toddlers specific foods that have a higher risk of aspiration such as peanuts, hot dogs, and whole grapes. The symptoms from a foreign body aspiration depend on the location and degree of obstruction but usually include recurrent and persistent cough, wheezing, and recurrent pneumonia or atelectasis in the same lobe of the lung. A foreign body is more likely to be aspirated into the right mainstem bronchus rather than the left, as its course is more vertical.

Pneumonia • When a segment of the lung is obstructed, bacterial pneumonia often results, most commonly caused by *S. pneumoniae* in otherwise healthy children. Group A *Streptococcus* is a common pathogen, however, it usually is limited to the upper airway causing exudative pharyngitis. *S. aureus* is an uncommon cause of pneumonia and results in a rapidly worsening clinical course, often with empyema. *M. pneumoniae* is a common pathogen in older adolescents and may cause symptoms ranging from wheezing with no lobar infiltrate to severe lobar pneumonia. *H. influenzae* type B is an uncommon pathogen as most children receive vaccination for this infection in infancy.

Diagnosis • Diagnosis of an aspirated foreign body can be difficult, especially if the object is radiolucent or not causing complete obstruction. Partial obstruction resulting in a "ball-valve" effect may cause overinflation of the distal lung segment. Complete obstruction causes atelectasis. X-ray findings with fluoroscopy reveal exaggerated shifting of the lungs and airways with inspiration and expiration as the obstructed area remains fixed in volume. However, if a foreign body is suspected and there are no findings on fluoroscopy, diagnosis may require CT scan of the lungs or bronchoscopy.

Wheezing • This has a wide differential diagnosis including recurrent reversible airway narrowing (asthma), increased fluid in the lungs (congestive heart disease or renal disease), external narrowing of an airway (vascular ring or mass effect), internal airway narrowing (foreign body aspiration or airway lesion such as papilloma), or infection (bronchiolitis or pneumonia). Croup classically causes upper airway narrowing and results in stridor, which is inspiratory, rather than wheezing, which is expiratory.

Answers • 1-A 2-B 3-E

CASE PRESENTATION

A 12-month-old boy presents with diarrhea. His mother reports that he has had intermittent diarrhea for the past several months with about four loose stools a day. She denies seeing any blood in the stools. He has a very good appetite and is still taking a bottle. He drinks several bottles a day of fruit juice but eats little solid food at regular meal times. His past medical history is significant for two previous episodes of otitis media but is otherwise negative. Family history is negative. On physical examination he is active and alert, sitting on his mother's lap drinking a bottle of juice. His length is 75 cm (25%), weight 8.4 kg (<5%), head circumference 47 cm (50%), heart rate 120/minute, and respiratory rate 20/minute. Physical examination is normal. Previous measurements are obtained and are plotted on the growth charts on the following two pages.

Laboratory testing reveals:

Neutrophil count	4000/ml
Platelet count	100,000/ml
Hemoglobin	10 g/dl
Hematocrit	30%
Stool hemoccult	negative
Urinalysis	specific gravity 1.005, pH 5 no protein/blood/glucose

1. What is the most likely cause of this child's poor growth?
   A. Hypothyroidism
   B. Growth hormone deficiency
   C. Inadequate nutrition
   D. Anemia
   E. Congenital malformation syndrome

2. What is the most efficient evaluation and/or treatment that should be considered as the next step in caring for this patient?
   A. Erythrocyte sedimentation rate
   B. Urine culture
   C. Prealbumin, albumin, ferritin, and folate levels
   D. Nutritional counseling and recheck weight
   E. Wrist x-ray to determine bone age

3. What is the most likely cause of the anemia in this child?
   A. Malabsorption
   B. Inadequate dietary iron
   C. Chronic blood loss
   D. Deficiency of intrinsic factor
   E. *Giardia* overgrowth in the terminal ileum

COMMENT

Failure to thrive (FTT) • FTT is a common diagnosis of infancy and childhood, indicating an inadequate weight gain with growth or weight loss. The different diagnoses that can lead to this condition are numerous but the approach is simple: evaluate the pattern of growth, take a careful history, and reevaluate closely with each intervention. For example, children with FTT due to inadequate nutrition present as is seen in this case, with a spared head circumference and a relatively less affected length than weight. Likewise the age of presentation is significant as FTT in early infancy is more likely to indicate a genetic or congenital defect while FTT occurring later is often caused by inadequate nutrition. Calories can be insufficient for growth if there is (1) inadequate intake, (2) malabsorption, or (3) increased demand as with a chronic illness. Inadequate intake may be caused by feeding difficulties, a diet deficient in calories and nutritional requirements, or vomiting/gastrointestinal reflux.

Fruit juice FTT • This has been recognized as a presentation of FTT in toddlers, usually those who are bottle addicts and carry their juice everywhere, drinking constantly throughout the day. These toddlers are satiated by this nutritionally inadequate "juice," actually usually a drink that is more sugar than fruit, and will not eat well at meal times. They drink an increasing amount of this simple sugar solution resulting in an osmotic diarrhea, iron deficiency anemia, and poor growth. If they drink their bottle at night while supine in bed, as they almost always do, they are also prone to recurrent otitis media and dental caries.

Evaluation • Evaluation of FTT can be extensive, chasing every possible diagnosis in the long differential. However this approach has been repeatedly demonstrated to be expensive and inefficient. Rather, laboratory testing should be directed by a careful history and physical examination with close patient reevaluation for expected response to interventions. If the most likely diagnosis is inadequate caloric intake then an intervention to change the diet with immediate documentation of weight gain can be both diagnostic and therapeutic.

Answers • 1-C 2-D 3-B

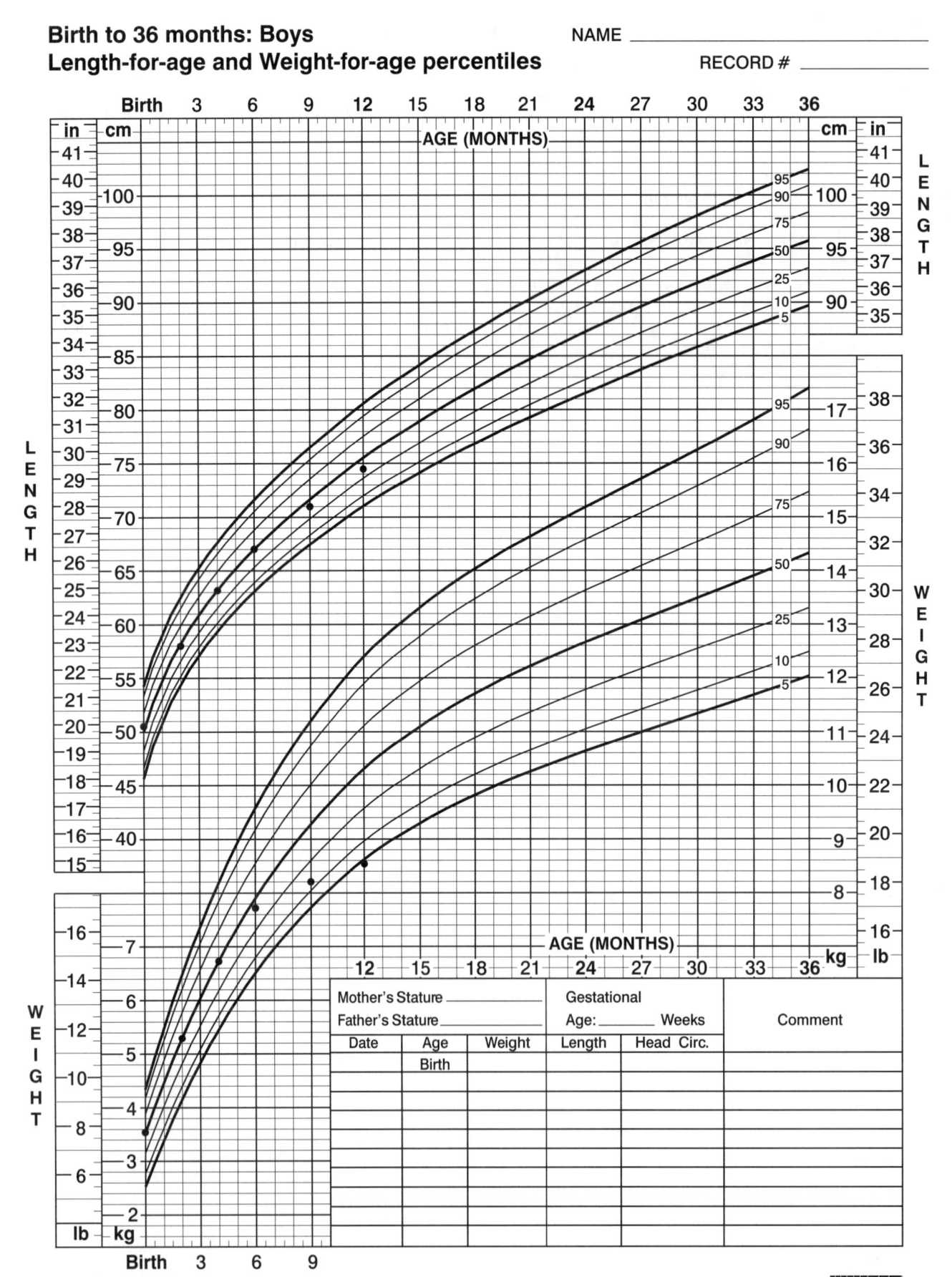

Birth to 36 months: Boys
Length-for-age and Weight-for-age percentiles

NAME _____
RECORD # _____

POOR GROWTH IN A TODDLER 43

**Birth to 36 months: Boys
Head circumference-for-age and
Weight-for-length percentiles**

NAME _____

RECORD # _____

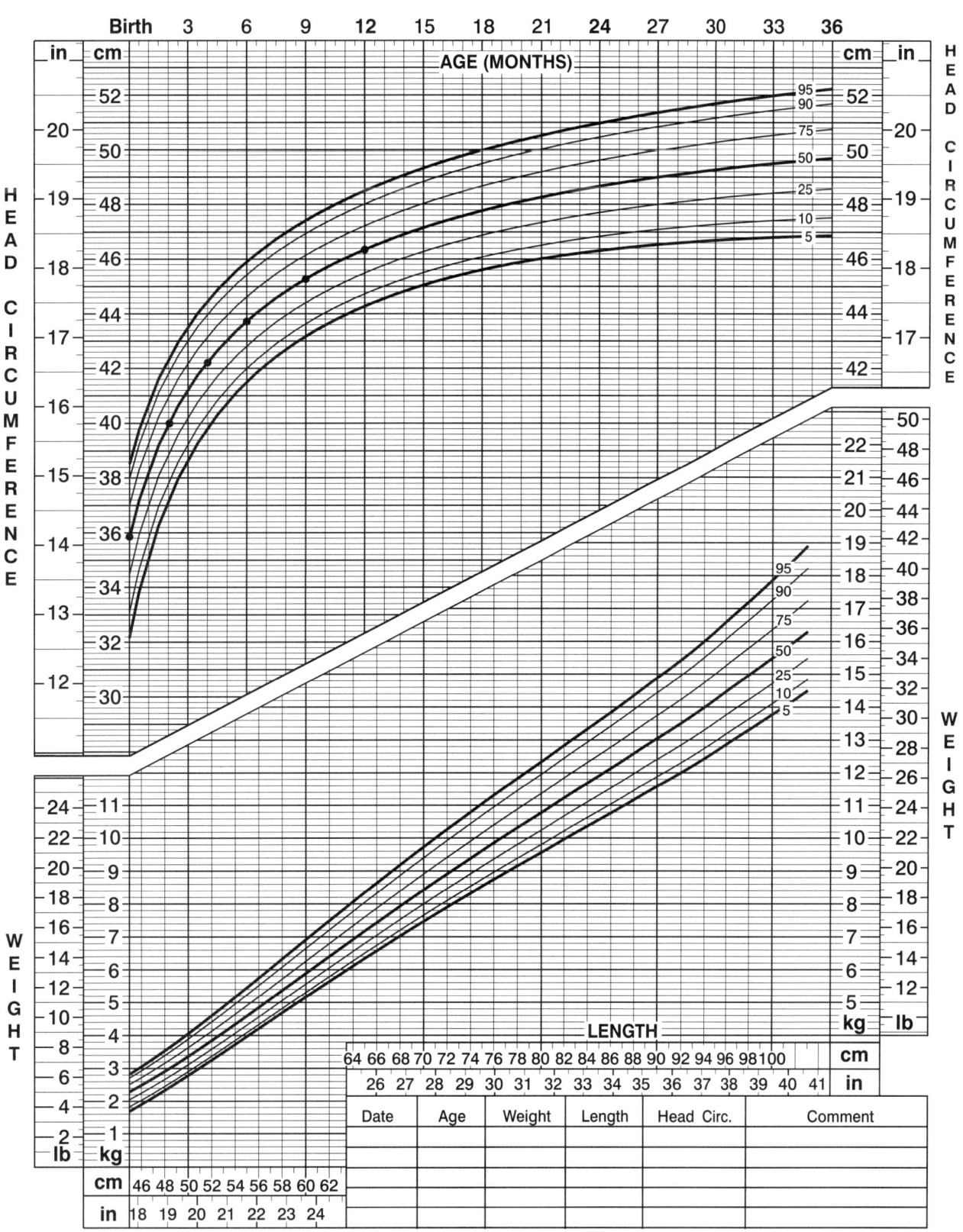

Published May 30, 2000 (modified 10/16/00).
SOURCE: Developed by the National Center for Health Statistics in collaboration with
the National Center for Chronic Disease Prevention and Health Promotion (2000).
http://www.cdc.gov/growthcharts

CDC
SAFER·HEALTHIER·PEOPLE™

DIARRHEA IN A TODDLER

CASE PRESENTATION

An 18-month-old child presents with fever, vomiting, and diarrhea. He was well until yesterday when he had a decreased appetite and vomited after eating lunch. His mother then noticed that he felt warm and found his temperature to be 102 degrees. Since then he has remained intermittently febrile despite acetaminophen every six hours, refuses to eat and drinks little of the milk and juice he has been offered, and has had about eight diapers with watery diarrhea, with no apparent blood. He is fussy and less active than usual. He attends daycare but his mother does not know of specific exposures to other illnesses. The family has well water and no pets in the home.

On physical examination he is irritable, crying but consolable by his mother, sitting in her lap. He does not produce tears with crying. His weight is 11 kg (50%) with a length of 80 cm (50%). Vital signs are: temperature 101.5 degrees, heart rate 120/minute, respiratory rate 20/minute, blood pressure 100/50 mmHg. Physical examination is normal.

1. What degree of dehydration, as a percent of body weight loss, would you estimate for this patient?
   A. <5%
   B. 5%
   C. 10%
   D. 15%
   E. 20%

2. What is the most likely diagnosis in this patient?
   A. *Giardia lamblia* gastroenteritis
   B. Milk allergy
   C. Congenital adrenal hyperplasia
   D. Rotavirus gastroenteritis
   E. *Shigella* gastroenteritis

3. What treatment would you recommend for this patient?
   A. Oral hydration with fruit juices or clear beverages
   B. Oral hydration with milk
   C. Intravenous hydration with one-quarter normal saline
   D. Oral hydration with electrolyte and glucose solution
   E. BRAT diet (bread, rice, applesauce, and toast)

COMMENT

Diarrhea • This is a symptom that includes not only stool change in consistency but also an increase in stool frequency. When combined with the symptom of vomiting the diagnosis is usually gastroenteritis. Worldwide, viral gastroenteritis is a leading cause of illness and death in young children, especially in countries with limited access to clean water and medical care. The clinical features of infectious gastroenteritis include abrupt onset of diarrhea, usually with fever and vomiting, after a short incubation period. Although not an absolutely reliable axiom, viral gastroenteritis usually causes lower fever than bacterial gastroenteritis and the diarrhea is not bloody. Symptoms of viral gastroenteritis should resolve over only a few days, with the only major complication being dehydration.

Dehydration • Dehydration in a young child can develop rapidly and be difficult to detect using the clinical signs seen in adults, such as hypotension and orthostatic changes, as a child's cardiovascular system maintains normal vital signs until reaching the edge of shock and accurate orthostatic measurements are all but impossible to obtain in a fussy child. Instead, clinical signs in children include frequency of urination (although this is difficult to ascertain when a child in diapers is having watery diarrhea), the presence of tears when crying, dry tacky buccal mucosa, sunken-appearing eyes, a sunken anterior fontanel, and abnormal skin turgor that remains tented after pinching. The clinical signs indicating a general assessment of the degree of dehydration (percent of body weight loss) in young children are listed in Table 6.

Etiology • Gastroenteritis in children is such a common condition that the full spectrum of underlying causes is often overlooked as the most likely etiology is viral infection, usually with either rotavirus or enteric adenovirus. Other etiologies include bacterial infections (*Shigella, Salmonella, Campylobacter, Clostridium*, or *E. coli*), parasitic infections (*Giardia* or *Entamoeba*), toxins such as heavy metal ingestion or the enterotoxins produced with staphylococcal food poisoning, endocrinopathies (thyrotoxicosis or congenital adrenal hyperplasia in salt-losing crisis), acute abdominal crisis (for example, malrotation with volvulus), or other illnesses such as inflammatory bowel disease. Although other diagnoses are never impossible, in this patient, an otherwise healthy toddler with acute onset of symptoms who is in daycare with the inevitable exposure to rotavirus and adenovirus, viral gastroenteritis is so likely that further evaluation is only indicated if he does not respond to treatment or has recurrent episodes.

Treatment • Treatment of viral gastroenteritis is supportive, to prevent dehydration or rehydrate from fluid losses. As water, electrolytes, and simple carbohydrates are still readily absorbed, oral hydration is indicated unless the patient is unable to tolerate oral fluids, the family is unable to adequately care for the child at home, or the patient has severe dehydration with electrolyte imbalance. Preparations used for oral rehydration should include electrolytes with adequate, but not excessive, carbohydrates. Fruit juices and soda beverages are just the opposite and their high osmolality due to a large sugar content may exacerbate the diarrheal losses by contributing to an osmotic diarrhea. Infants can resume breast feeding as soon as they are able and older children can resume feeding as tolerated. Often after gastroenteritis, children do better on a diet that is low in fat and complex carbohydrates such as the BRAT diet. A vaccination developed for rotavirus has not been recommended for use as it has been associated with an increased risk of intussusception.

TABLE 6 • Signs of Dehydration

Clinical Sign	<5%	5%	≥10%
Wet diapers	Normal to ↓	↓	↓
General appearance	Alert	Fussy	Lethargic
Tears	Normal	None	None
Buccal mucosa	Normal	Normal	Dry
Skin turgor	Normal	Normal	Tents

Answers • 1-B 2-D 3-D

CASE PRESENTATION

A 5-year-old boy presents for his annual physical examination. He is well with no complaints at this time. He does have a past medical history of asthma and was hospitalized several months ago with severe status asthmaticus. His current medications are a steroid inhaler used daily with occasional use of an albuterol inhaler for wheezing, averaging about twice a week. He has had no other medical illnesses. He will be enrolled in kindergarten this fall. Physical examination is normal. His previous immunizations are listed in Table 7.

1. What additional vaccinations would most schools require for a 5-year-old with this immunization record?
   A. DTaP #5, MMR #2, and pneumococcal
   B. DTaP #5, MMR #2, and IPV
   C. DTaP #5, MMR #2, and hepatitis B #4
   D. DTaP #5, MMR #2, and Hib #5
   E. MMR #2, dT, and Hib #5

2. What additional vaccinations should be considered for this patient?
   A. Influenza and varicella
   B. Oral polio and varicella
   C. Pneumococcal heptavalent conjugate vaccine (PCV) and varicella
   D. Inactivated polio and hepatitis A
   E. Influenza and inactivated polio

3. Children with which of the following conditions should receive pneumococcal heptavalent conjugate vaccine (PCV)?
   A. Severe asthma
   B. Age under 23 months
   C. Congenital heart disease
   D. Afterschool care for elementary school-age children
   E. Prematurity

4. Oral polio vaccine should be used in which situation?
   A. Patients with an immunocompromised family member
   B. Patients who are immunocompromised
   C. Oral polio vaccine is not indicated for use in the United States
   D. Patients with malabsorption
   E. Patients with a history of febrile seizures

COMMENT

Immunizations • Immunizations have had a profound effect on the health of children, virtually eliminating infectious diseases that were once common causes of childhood morbidity and mortality. The nationwide, coordinated effort to develop a vaccination for polio funded by dimes collected from children themselves, the March of Dimes, and culminating in community vaccination programs throughout the United States in the 1950s remains one of the most dramatic stories of medicine. Reviewing a patient's immunization needs at each well-child examination is an important aspect of preventive care. As infants have relatively poorer immune response to antigens, repeated vaccinations must be administered for several doses. Vaccines can contain live virus that has been altered to lessen its virulence (attenuated, live vaccine such as MMR), killed virus (IPV), or an extracted toxoid (tetanus). Repeated exposure to a vaccine results in a greater immune response with each dose.

Required routine vaccination • For a 4- to 6-year-old child, required routine vaccinations include completing the age-appropriate series for hepatitis B, DTaP, IPV, and MMR. As polio has been essentially eliminated and exposure to wild virus is less likely than the risk of disease following use of the live oral polio vaccine, only IPV is used in the United States. Younger children should have been protected by Hib and PCV, however, if these series are not complete, further vaccination in the older child is not indicated as *Haemophilus influenzae* Type B and pneumococcus are no longer devastating pathogens beyond early childhood in normal children. Vaccination with varicella is recommended at age 12 months or older if the child has not already had chicken pox, however, this vaccination is not always a requirement by school systems.

Special indications • Special indications for vaccination include protection for medically fragile children or those in an environment that might expose them to illness. Influenza vaccination is recommended each fall for children with many different chronic illnesses, including moderate or severe asthma. Children with immunologic disorders or asplenia who have an increased risk of pneumococcal disease should receive pneumoccal vaccination beyond the routinely recommended age and should receive additional protection with pneumococcal polysaccharide vaccine if at very high risk. Children living in conditions with a high rate of exposure to hepatitis A should receive that vaccination series.

TABLE 7 • Age

Vaccine	Birth	2 months	4 months	6 months	12 months	18 months
Hepatitis B	✓	✓		✓		
DTaP		✓	✓	✓		✓
IPV		✓	✓		✓	
Hib		✓	✓	✓	✓	
MMR					✓	

DTaP = diphtheria, tetanus, and acellular pertussis.
Hib = *Haemophilus influenzae* Type B.
MMR = measles, mumps, and rubella.
IPV = inactivated polio.

Answers • 1-B 2-A 3-B 4-C

FEVER AND RASH IN A PRESCHOOL CHILD

● CASE PRESENTATION

A 4-year-old girl presents with a rash and fever for the past seven days. She has had fever up to 105 degrees, with little response to acetaminophen. Her rash initially just involved her hands and feet with generalized redness, but the skin on her fingers has now started peeling. Her mother also states that she has been very irritable, refuses to eat and drinks little, and has had red, swollen eyes. Two days ago an emergency department physician diagnosed left otitis media and treated her with high-dose amoxicillin (80 mg/kg/d). Since then she has not improved. Review of symptoms is otherwise negative with no cough, pulling on her ears, diarrhea, vomiting, or rhinorrhea. Family history is positive for penicillin allergy.

On physical examination her weight and height are 50% for age. Vital signs are temperature 104.5 degrees, heart rate 120/minute, respiratory rate 30/minute, blood pressure 110/70 mmHg. She is sitting on her mother's lap, crying tears, and is very irritable when moved by her mother or approached. Physical examination is significant for swollen, erythematous lips, hands and feet, small sheets of skin peeling from the distal fingers and toes, injected conjunctiva with no exudate, erythematous tympanic membranes bilaterally with decreased mobility, and bilateral cervical lymphadenopathy. The rest of her physical examination is normal.

1. Which diagnosis is unlikely in this patient?
   A. Toxic shock syndrome
   B. Scarlet fever
   C. Stevens-Johnson syndrome
   D. Kawasaki disease
   E. Acute bacterial endocarditis

2. What laboratory results do you expect to find in this patient to confirm the most likely diagnosis?
   A. Positive throat culture
   B. Positive blood culture
   C. Diagnostic dermatopathologic findings on skin biopsy
   D. Thrombocytosis
   E. Hypernatremia

3. Possible complications of this illness include:
   A. Myocarditis
   B. Pyelonephritis
   C. Pancreatitis
   D. Seizure
   E. Cellulitis

4. Treatment should include:
   A. Acetaminophen
   B. Intravenous immune globulin
   C. Antibiotic coverage of resistant group A *streptococcus*
   D. Transfusion
   E. High-dose steroids

● COMMENT

Kawasaki disease • This is a perplexing disease usually seen in preschool children. The diagnosis remains purely clinical, based on specific criteria (listed in Table 8), and confirmed with expected laboratory results such as marked thrombocytosis, elevated sedimentation rate, hyponatremia, and sterile pyuria. Other associated clinical findings may include aseptic meningitis, arthritis, hydrops of the gallbladder, mild hepatitis, and apparent otitis media. The most significant complication is myocarditis that may result in coronary artery aneurysms.

Differential diagnosis • Differential diagnosis of Kawasaki disease is of necessity extensive, as this is a diagnosis of exclusion. Illnesses that may have similar clinical features include scarlet fever, toxic shock syndrome, drug reactions such as Stevens-Johnson syndrome, and autoimmune diseases. Careful history and examination can find distinguishing features. For example, the desquamation in scarlet fever begins centrally rather than with the fingertips and occurs with tiny, sand like flakes of skin rather than larger pieces. Toxic shock syndrome usually has rapid onset of multiorgan involvement. Stevens-Johnson syndrome and drug sensitivity rashes usually progress fairly rapidly and often include vesicular lesions, a feature not consistent with Kawasaki disease.

Treatment • Treatment of Kawasaki disease includes a dose of intravenous immune globulin (2 g/kg) with high-dose aspirin (80–100 mg/kg/d) until the acute phase of illness has ended. In fact, response to treatment should be immediate and the diagnosis may be questioned if the patient does not defervesce and become less irritable within one or two days. Lower-dose aspirin (3 to 5 mg/kg/d) should be continued for at least six to eight weeks during convalescence. Long-term follow-up includes monitoring for coronary artery aneurysms.

TABLE 8 • Diagnostic Criteria for Kawasaki Disease

Fever lasting for at least five days
Illness not explained by any other diagnosis
Presence of at least four of the following signs
1. Bilateral bulbar conjunctival injection, usually nonpurulent
2. Mucous membrane changes of the oropharynx
3. Changes of the peripheral extremities such as edema/erythema in the acute phase or desquamation in the subacute phase
4. Rash, usually truncal, polymorphous but nonvesicular
5. Cervical adenopathy ≥1.5 cm

Answers • 1-E 2-D 3-A 4-B

CASE PRESENTATION

A 17-year-old girl presents for a routine yearly physical examination with no complaints except chronic fatigue. She does not eat well, usually does not finish a meal, but denies a desire to lose weight or purging. Of further review of symptoms she does reveal that occasionally her wrists and knees ache and that she has not had menarche. The rest of her history is negative. She is an excellent student with no risk-taking behaviors and no sexual activity. On physical examination she is 152 cm tall (<5%), with a weight of 40 kg (<5%) and a body mass index of 17 (<5%). She has slight abdominal tenderness of the right lower quadrant with palpation and several tender, erythematous raised lesions on both legs but otherwise her physical examination is normal with secondary sexual characteristics of Tanner stage 4 breast development and Tanner stage 3 pubic hair development. Initial laboratory tests include:

Complete blood count:	
Hematocrit	30%
Hemoglobin	10 g/dl
White blood count	6000/mm^3
Platelet count	500,000/mm^3
Erythrocyte sedimentation rate	70 mm/h
Albumin	2.0 g/dl (normal 3.5 to 4.8)
Follicle stimulating hormone	2.5 mIU/ml (normal 3.0 to 20.0)
Luteinizing hormone	2.0 mIU/ml (normal 5 to 150)
Thyroid stimulating hormone	<0.50 μIU/ml (normal 0.5 to 5.0)
Urinalysis	Normal

1. Given the history and laboratory test results in this patient, which diagnosis can be eliminated?
   A. Malignancy
   B. Inflammatory bowel disease
   C. Anorexia nervosa
   D. Appendiceal abscess
   E. Juvenile rheumatoid arthritis

2. What additional evaluation/treatment is indicated at this time?
   A. Nutritional counseling and follow weight gain over the next three months
   B. Rectal examination and hemoccult
   C. Biopsy skin lesions
   D. Psychiatric evaluation and counseling
   E. Bone marrow aspirate

3. The primary amenorrhea seen in this patient is most likely caused by:
   A. Hypothyroidism
   B. Anemia
   C. Chronic illness
   D. Hypogonadism
   E. Depression

COMMENT

Inflammatory bowel disease (IBD) • IBD can present at any time of life but usually presents in adolescence or adulthood and often with a series of gradually accumulating, confusing symptoms that in retrospect can be tied together to make the diagnosis. In adolescents, growth failure affecting both weight and height may precede overt clinical symptoms by several years, sometimes also causing a delay in pubertal development as in this patient with primary amenorrhea and growth failure. The anorexia is gradual, sometimes developing in a subconscious response to abdominal pain, and families become accustomed to the child's eating patterns over time without realizing the impact. As IBD is a disorder of inflammation, the extragastrointestinal symptoms are numerous and may include arthritis, skin lesions (erythema nodosum), digital clubbing, and renal or biliary stones. Blood loss may result in anemia. Malnutrition and hypoalbuminemia may result from enteric protein loss, poor intake, and malabsorption. The two most common types of IBD, Crohn disease and ulcerative colitis, differ in the areas of the bowel they affect, with ulcerative colitis usually limited to the colon and Crohn disease occurring anywhere throughout the gastrointestinal tract, often with normal bowel separating affected areas (skip lesions), and may be transmural with development of fistulas. In adolescent girls, IBD often presents as amenorrhea, primary or secondary. This may be caused by several possible mechanisms including malnutrition, either by being significantly underweight or by being under 17% total body fat, or simply by the effect of any serious chronic illness affecting the hypothalamus.

Differential diagnosis • Differential diagnosis for a patient with IBD is extensive, especially as it usually presents with a confusing constellation of symptoms. The differential diagnosis for primary amenorrhea and poor weight gain in an adolescent girl includes anorexia nervosa. In this patient, anorexia nervosa can be eliminated as the DSM IV criteria are not met (there is no desire to lose weight) and there is an elevated erythrocyte sedimentation rate. The other diagnoses, malignancy especially lymphoma, abdominal abscess such as a ruptured appendiceal abscess, and other inflammatory illnesses such as juvenile rheumatoid arthritis, are all possible. In addition, a complete differential diagnosis may include infections (such as *Yersinia enterocolitica*) or forms of vasculitis (such as systemic lupus erythematosis).

Evaluation • Evaluation of a patient with possible IBD should always start with a thorough history and physical examination, as with all complicated patients. In a patient with abdominal complaints this must include a rectal examination with testing for occult blood loss. Rectal examination with abdominal palpation can detect lower abdominal masses not felt on routine abdominal examination, especially those that are hiding behind the cecum. Further evaluation usually includes radiographic studies and endoscopy.

Answers • 1-C   2-B   3-C

CASE PRESENTATION

A 12-year-old boy presents with knee pain for two months. His pain is located in both knees and increases in severity in the evening such that he has difficulty sleeping. He also complains of a sore knot on both knees. He had trauma recently when he was kicked in the lower leg during a soccer game but was wearing a shin guard. He otherwise is well with a good appetite and no weight loss. He is very active and plays on a soccer team throughout the year. On physical examination he has a height of 145 cm (25%) with a weight of 30 kg (5%) and vital signs including a heart rate 68/minute, blood pressure 100/60 and respiratory rate 20/minute. Physical examination is significant for pubertal development of genitalia Tanner stage 3, pubic hair Tanner stage 2, and 2 × 2 cm tender elevated areas on both legs below the patella.

1. The most likely diagnosis in this patient is:
   A. Osteogenic sarcoma
   B. Stress fractures
   C. Osteomyelitis
   D. Osgood-Schlatter disease
   E. Patellofemoral syndrome

2. Treatment for this patient should include:
   A. Rest and decreased soccer participation
   B. Ice
   C. Knee immobilization
   D. Steroid medication
   E. A, B, and C

3. Factors that contribute to this condition include:
   A. Female gender
   B. Rapid change in height
   C. Family history of arthritis
   D. Lateral deviation of the patella with movement
   E. Underweight body habitus

COMMENT

Knee pain • In a child and adolescent, knee pain may indicate pathology in the knee itself or may be caused by referred pain from the hip. For this reason the differential diagnosis of knee pain is extensive but may include trauma (effusion, ligamentous injury, or fracture), infection (septic arthritis or osteomyelitis), malignancy (osteogenic sarcoma, Ewing's sarcoma, or benign bone tumors), metabolic disorders (rickets), or overuse/sports injuries (patellofemoral syndromes or Osgood-Schlatter disease).

Osgood-Schlatter disease • This is a common problem, especially in very active, rapidly growing boys during early puberty. At this stage of maximal height velocity, the muscles and tendons literally cannot stretch fast enough to accommodate the area of the body with the greatest growth rate, the knees. The constant pull on the insertion of the patellar tendon results in microfractures of the tibial tubercle area of the epiphysis, causing it to be elevated and tender. Radiographs reveal this elevation and sometimes a separation of the tibial tuberosity in severe cases. Treatment is simply to reduce the stress on this site while the child continues growing by resting the leg and reducing physical exercise that maximize the use of the quadriceps. Nonsteroidal anti-inflammatory medication may alleviate some of the pain. Immobilization of the knee may be necessary but rarely is surgery indicated.

Answers • 1-D 2-E 3-B

CASE PRESENTATION

A 12-year-old girl presents for a yearly physical examination. Her mother is concerned that she has not yet had menses and that she has developed a white vaginal discharge for the last four months. The discharge varies in amount but is never heavy. She denies itching, genital lesions or rash, abdominal pain, or vaginal bleeding. On further confidential history, the patient denies sexual activity. Physical examination reveals a height of 147 cm (25%), weight 43 kg (50%), and normal vital signs. Secondary sexual characteristics include breasts Tanner stage 4 and pubic hair Tanner stage 3. Genital examination reveals normal female genitalia with a small amount of opaque thick vaginal discharge. The rest of the physical examination is normal.

1. Primary amenorrhea can be defined as lack of menarche by what age?
   A. 12 years
   B. 14 years
   C. 15 years
   D. 16 years
   E. 18 years

2. What is the most likely etiology of this patient's vaginal discharge?
   A. Gonoccocal cervicitis
   B. Chlamydial cervicitis
   C. Yeast vaginitis
   D. Physiologic leukorrhea
   E. Bacterial vaginosis

3. When counseling this patient and her mother about what they should expect over the next year, you explain that:
   A. She will not grow any taller and should start her menses within the next six months
   B. She will continue a rapid height velocity until beginning her menses and then continue to grow for the next one and a half years but with a gradually decreasing velocity
   C. She will continue a rapid height velocity until two years after menarche
   D. She will have menarche about age 16 and will grow until then

COMMENT

Puberty • Puberty is a time of rapid growth with changes in sexual development, cognitive development, and social development all occurring simultaneously. The result can be overwhelming confusion and trepidation on the part of both the adolescent and the parents! "Is my child's development normal?" is a common question asked of physicians during these years and therefore knowledge of normal development and when to look further into abnormal development is crucial. Puberty usually occurs at an earlier age in girls than in boys and is completed over a shorter interval in girls than in boys. The first sign of puberty in girls is thelarche followed within several months by adrenarche. In boys, testicular enlargement occurs first followed by development of pubic hair. Menarche occurs at an average age of about 12 to 13 years old although menarche is not deemed delayed until age 16.

Physiologic leukorrhea • This is a normal increase in vaginal mucous production in response to estrogen. Exposure to estrogen results in thickening and keritinization of the vaginal epithelium. These normal squamous epithelial cells may be seen on a "wet prep." In addition, the presence of lactobacillus in the vaginal flora, creating an acid pH, further indicates normal response to estrogen. Vaginal or cervical infections (such as gonorrhea or chlamydia) would reveal increased leukocytes on wet prep. Clue cells and an alkaline vaginal pH are the diagnostic features of bacterial vaginosis. Budding yeast or hyphae, especially seen on KOH prep, are seen with yeast vaginosis.

Growth • Growth during puberty accelerates rapidly. With girls, the height velocity increases until a peak that ends with menarche. Following menarche, growth continues for about one and a half years but at a gradually decreasing rate. Boys have a longer period of growth with a more gradual deceleration toward the end of puberty.

Answers • 1-D   2-D   3-B

RESPIRATORY DISTRESS IN A NEONATE

CASE PRESENTATION

A premature male infant presents with increasing respiratory distress at 6 hours of age. He was born at 28 weeks gestation after a pregnancy complicated only by a lack of prenatal care and precipitous vaginal delivery. At birth he was appropriate for gestational age with a normal physical examination and Apgar scores of 5 at one minute but increasing to 7 by five minutes after initial resuscitation with warming and stimulation. He was noted to have tachypnea at 4 hours of age that has gradually worsened. On physical examination he has a heart rate of 180/minute, respiratory rate of 80/minute, and is afebrile. He is grunting with expiration and has accessory muscle use, nasal flaring, and intracostal retractions with inspiration. His hands and feet are cyanotic and he is diffusely hypotonic.

1. What is the most likely etiology of this patient's respiratory distress?
   A. Group B streptococcal sepsis
   B. Cyanotic congenital heart disease
   C. Diaphragmatic hernia
   D. Hyaline membrane disease
   E. Congenital lobar emphysema

2. What results on diagnostic tests would confirm this diagnosis?
   A. Chest x-ray with ground glass appearance
   B. Neutropenia
   C. Hyponatremia
   D. Positive blood culture
   E. Metabolic alkalosis

3. Which characteristic is associated with an increased risk of this condition?
   A. Female gender
   B. African-American ethnic origin
   C. Infant of a diabetic mother
   D. Family history of emphysema
   E. Maternal smoking

4. Which treatment is not indicated in the initial care of this patient?
   A. Warmed ambient environment
   B. Mechanical ventilation with increased oxygen
   C. Endotracheal exogenous surfactant
   D. Bronchodilators
   E. Intravenous nutrition

COMMENT

Respiratory distress syndrome (hyaline membrane disease) (RDS)
• RDS is a common cause of mortality in otherwise normal premature infants, usually in those babies born before 36 weeks gestation, before their endogenous surfactant has coated the surface of their lungs. Without this lipid lining to reduce surface tension, the lungs of premature infants continue collapsing with each breath. Although they may sometimes appear normal at birth, this increased work of breathing and accumulating alveolar atelectasis soon causes the infant to have severe distress, hypoxemia, and respiratory failure. Besides the association with prematurity, RDS is more likely with male gender, Caucasian race, cesarean section delivery, twin pregnancies, and in infants born to diabetic mothers.

Differential diagnosis • Differential diagnosis includes many respiratory and cardiac illnesses. Infants born after a precipitous vaginal delivery or a cesarean delivery may have transient tachypnea of the newborn, with increased fluid in the lungs that rapidly resolves. Group B streptococcal sepsis can have a clinical presentation that is truly indistinguishable from RDS and must always be considered, especially in full-term infants with respiratory distress. Congenital heart disease usually differs in that there may be relatively normal lung fields but an abnormal cardiac shadow on x-ray. Congenital malformations of the lungs such as lobar emphysema usually have a distinctive hyperinflated segmental appearance. Diaphragmatic hernia will present with bowel in the chest on x-ray and a scaffoid abdomen.

Clinical presentation • Clinical presentation includes the increasing respiratory distress in the first day or two of life with tachypnea, nasal flaring, retractions (abdominal and intracostal), and peripheral cyanosis. In an attempt to reinflate their atelectatic lungs, patients have a distinctive grunting with respiration, usually in the expiratory phase. Chest x-ray has a diffuse, finely reticular appearance that has been described as "ground glass." Arterial blood gas reveals hypoxemia, hypercapnea and respiratory acidosis that may progress to metabolic acidosis in severely ill patients.

Treatment • Treatment is supportive with increased oxygen, often with continuous positive airway pressure (CPAP) or mechanical ventilation, decreased work of breathing by warming the ambient environment, minimized stress and handling of the patient, and adequate intravenous nutrition. The underlying deficiency of surfactant can be treated by endotracheal administration of exogenous surfactant.

Answers • 1-D 2-A 3-C 4-D

CASE PRESENTATION

An 18-month-old boy presents with intermittent outward deviation of his right eye. His mother has noticed it several times a week over the last month, usually in the late afternoon or evening. He is otherwise asymptomatic. Past medical history and family history are negative. On physical examination he is appropriate size with normal vital signs. Hirschberg corneal reflex test is normal. The alternate cover test reveals realignment to the midline from lateral deviation of the right eye when uncovered. Pupils are round and reactive to light with normal fundoscopic examinations.

1. The condition diagnosed by these findings on physical examination is:
   A. Pseudostrabismus
   B. Esotropia of the right eye
   C. Exotropia of the right eye
   D. Esotropia of the left eye
   E. Exotropia of the left eye

2. The next step in treatment or evaluation of this patient should be:
   A. Close reevaluation and further evaluation if the condition persists
   B. Evaluation of visual acuity
   C. Referral for further treatment
   D. Computed tomography of the optic muscles and optic nerve
   E. No further treatment is necessary

3. The Hirschberg corneal reflex test and cover tests should be performed on physical examinations in:
   A. Routine yearly well-child examinations in preschool children
   B. School-age children with abnormal vision screens
   C. Infants with unilateral white pupil
   D. Children with ocular trauma
   E. Children with conjunctivitis

COMMENT

Strabismus • Strabismus usually presents in preschool children, often with an eye that turns in or out with fatigue or when fixating on a distant object. Mothers notice a deviated eye at the end of the day when the child is tired. As with many conditions in children, early diagnosis is essential to prevent serious consequences such as amblyopia or "lazy eye" as one eye is used preferentially over the other. For this reason, screening for strabismus should be a part of the well-child examination of preschool children with the Hirschberg corneal reflex test (symmetric or asymmetric location of the light reflex in the corneas) for fixed strabismus and the cover tests (deviation and realignment with covering and uncovering) for intermittent strabismus. Esotropia (inward deviation of the eye) is more common than exotropia (outward deviation) although pseudostrabismus (false appearance of eye deviation often due to epicanthal folds) is more common than either.

Evaluation and treatment • These should be instituted even if visual acuity can be documented to be normal, although vision testing in a preschool child is a challenge and often inaccurate in the pediatric office setting. Early detection and simple patching of the "good" eye can prevent amblyopia. Patients with strabismus should be referred to a pediatric ophthalmologist for further detailed testing and treatment.

Answers • 1-C 2-C 3-A

DEHYDRATION IN A CHILD

● CASE PRESENTATION

A 9-month-old boy has diarrhea. He weighs 10 kilograms and other significant physical exam findings include: sunken anterior fontanel, lethargy, dry mucous membranes, poor skin turgor, blood pressure 65/45 mmHg, pulse 150 beats/min, and respiratory rate 32 breaths/min.

1. You decide he is severely dehydrated and requires immediate volume expansion. Of the following, the MOST appropriate volume of normal saline to be administered as a bolus is:
   A. 50 ml
   B. 500 ml
   C. 1000 ml
   D. 200 ml
   E. 0 ml

2. Before the normal saline is started, he develops generalized tonic-clonic seizures. His sodium level is 115 mEq/dl, but glucose and calcium levels are normal. The best treatment would be intravenous administration of:
   A. Calcium chloride
   B. Glucose
   C. Hypertonic saline
   D. Normal saline
   E. Phenobarbitol

3. Appropriate treatment is initiated and the seizures stop. You calculate his sodium and fluid deficits, maintenance requirements, and estimate ongoing losses. Which of the following statements is not true?
   A. Maintenance sodium requirements are 3–5 mEq/kg of body weight
   B. The serum sodium level should be normalized as quickly as possible to avoid further seizures
   C. Maintenance fluid requirements are 1500 ml/m^2
   D. The degree of fluid deficit is equal to the amount of acute weight loss or it can be estimated by the degree of clinical dehydration
   E. Tachypnea, fever, and burns increase maintenance fluid requirements

4. You admit him to the hospital. After six hours in the hospital you become concerned because his diapers are dry and no urine is obtained on catheterization. His blood urea nitrogen is 50 mEq/dl and his creatinine is 1.1 mEq/dl. After reexamining the child, you suspect the cause of his kidney failure is prerenal. Which one of the following tests would you order next?
   A. Fractional excretion of sodium
   B. Renal angiography
   C. Echocardiogram
   D. Chest x-ray
   E. Serum albumin

● COMMENT

Dehydration • Dehydration is common in children with gastrointestinal illness, but it is usually mild and can be treated as an outpatient. The physical signs of moderate and severe dehydration in children include: dry mucous membranes, lack of tears, sunken eyes or fontanel, lethargy, tachycardia, hypotension, decreased urine output, and poor skin turgor. In severe dehydration, such as this child, the intravascular volume must be restored to stabilize the vital signs. This can be achieved with a 20 ml/kg intravenous bolus of normal saline or lactated Ringer's solution administered over 30 to 60 minutes. If shock is present, the fluids should be administered at a more rapid rate. Intravenous fluid therapy must include deficit replacement, maintenance requirements, and replacement of ongoing losses. Maintenance requirements are 3–5 mEq/L for sodium and 1500 ml/m^2 for fluid. Maintenance requirements for fluids can be estimated by using the "100/50/20 rule": for the first 0–10 kg of body weight, 100 cc/kg of fluid is required each 24 hours; for next 10 kg of body weight (11–20 kg), an additional 50 cc/kg of fluid is required; and for any weight greater than 20 kg, an additional 20 cc/kg of fluid is required. For example, an 8 kg child requires 100 ml/kg of fluid for maintenance in 24 hours, which equals 800 ml/24 hours. A 20 kg child requires 100 ml/kg for the first 10 kg (1000 cc) plus 50 ml/kg for the next 10 kg (500 cc), which equals 1500 ml of maintenance fluid required in 24 hours. A 24 kg child requires 100 ml/kg for the first 10 kg (1000 cc), 50 ml/kg for the next 10 kg (500 cc), and 20 ml/kg for any weight above 20 kg (80 ml), which equals 1580 ml of maintenance fluids required in 24 hours. Maintenance fluid requirements are increased in the face of fever, increased skin or respiratory tract losses, and catabolic states.

Hyponatremia • This is the result of greater losses of sodium than water in the diarrhea. It can also be caused in infants by the ingestion of dilute formula or can be present in infants with congenital adrenal hyperplasia. Infants are predisposed to develop hyponatremia because of their limited ability to excrete free water due to a low glomerular filtration rate. Central nervous system symptoms (apathy, lethargy, listlessness, agitation, vomiting, and seizures) can develop when the serum sodium concentration falls below 120 mEq/L. A bolus of 5 ml/kg of 3% saline administered over 10 to 20 minutes increases the serum sodium concentration by 4 to 5 mEq/L, which usually is sufficient to control the seizures. Anticonvulsant medications such as phenobarbitol or lorazepam could be administered, but multiple doses may be required and this treatment does not address the underlying etiology of the seizures.

Prerenal failure • This is a complication of severe dehydration. In the face of oliguric renal failure an elevated blood urea nitrogen to creatinine ratio greater than 20:1 and fractional excretion of sodium (FENa) less than 1 are indicative of prerenal failure. The FENa calculation is (urine sodium divided by plasma sodium) divided by (urine creatinine divided by plasma creatinine) multiplied by 100. Prerenal states should resolve with aggressive fluid resuscitation.

Answers • 1-D 2-C 3-B 4-A

CASE PRESENTATION

A 4-year-old previously healthy white male presents with a three-day history of abdominal pain and bloody diarrhea. His mother and 6-year-old sister had similar complaints but their symptoms have resolved. He has not had any emesis or fever and his diarrhea is resolving. He has had only sips of fluids over the last 24 hours and has not had any urine output in twelve hours. He has become increasingly irritable at times and is only consolable by his mother. On physical examination, he is tachycardic, but his other vital signs are stable. He is lying quietly in his mother's arms, but cries when approached for examination. He does not have tears, his mucous membranes are dry, and his eyes are sunken. His cardiac examination is significant for a grade III/VI systolic ejection murmur at the left sternal border. His abdomen has active bowel sounds but is minimally tender to deep palpation diffusely. He has no hepatosplenomegaly. His examination is otherwise unremarkable. Laboratory evaluation is significant for a creatinine of 5.7 mg/dl. His hemoglobin is 5 g/dl, white blood cell count is 7000/ml, and his platelet count is 5000/ml.

1. You suspect hemolytic uremic syndrome (HUS). If you are correct, the peripheral smear must show which of the following findings?
   A. Spherocytosis
   B. At least 20% lymphoblasts
   C. Microcytic hypochromia
   D. Fragmented red blood cells and burr cells
   E. Eosinophilia

2. Which is the most likely cause of hemolytic uremic syndrome in this case?
   A. Tuberculosis
   B. *Streptococcus pneumoniae*
   C. Rotavirus
   D. *Escherichia coli* O157:H7
   E. Epstein-Barr virus

3. Acceptable treatment options for hemolytic uremic syndrome include:
   A. Dialysis
   B. Packed red blood cell and platelet transfusions
   C. Aggressive enteral or parenteral nutritional support
   D. Antibiotic therapy for the underlying colitis
   E. A, B, and C

4. Known exposures to the *E. coli* O157:H7 include:
   A. Undercooked hamburger
   B. Daycare
   C. Unpasturized milk
   D. Inadequately chlorinated pools
   E. All of the above

COMMENT

Hemolytic-uremic syndrome • The findings of bloody diarrhea followed by lethargy and pallor suggests the diagnosis of hemolytic-uremic syndrome (HUS). Respiratory distress may occur as a result of fluid overload or metabolic acidosis in association with acute renal failure. Findings on peripheral blood smear in HUS typically include thrombocytopenia as well as helmet cells, burr cells, and fragmented red blood cells. These abnormal red blood cell forms provide evidence of a microangiopathic hemolytic anemia. In the United States, HUS preceded by a diarrheal prodrome is most likely caused by an enterohemorrhagic strain of *Escherichia coli* called *E. coli* O157:H7. It produces a toxin that causes endothelial cell injury which results in the formation of microthrombi in the kidney and other organs, subsequent shearing of red blood cells, and renal failure. Exposure to the enterohemmorrhagic *E. coli* can be from undercooked hamburger, unpasteurized milk, or fecal-oral spread at home, in daycares, or in inadequately chlorinated pools. HUS has also been associated with a strain of *Streptococcus pneumoniae* that produces neuraminidase. Affected children often present with pneumonia without diarrhea and have a worse overall prognosis than those with a diarrheal prodome.

Treatment and prognosis • Treatment is with aggressive supportive care. This includes control of hypertension, nutritional support, packed red blood cell transfusions, fluid and electrolyte management, platelet transfusions for active bleeding, and dialysis if indicated. Treatment of the underlying colitis with antibiotics is not indicated, and theoretically could worsen the course if it resulted in a sudden burst of toxin release. Although the majority of children with HUS recover, some die during the acute disease from electrolyte imbalance and renal failure, hypertension-related problems, bleeding (particularly cerebral), or, rarely, cardiac involvement.

Answers • 1-D 2-D 3-E 4-E

CASE PRESENTATION

A 4-year-old male presents with the chief complaint of generalized swelling for one week. He had presented one week prior to this visit with cough, clear rhinorrhea, and facial swelling. He was diagnosed with allergic rhinitis and was treated with an antihistamine. Over the following week the swelling is his face increased and he developed swelling in his legs and hands. On further history, he has had decreased urine output but no gross hematuria. His appetite and activity are decreased. On physical examination his weight is increased by 8 pounds compared to the previous week. His pulse is 96 beats/minute, respiratory rate is 32 breaths/minute, and his blood pressure is 100/60 mmHg. He has marked periorbital and facial edema. His breath sounds are equal and clear. His abdomen is distended with active bowel sounds and a fluid wave. His scrotum is tennis-ball size, but not erythematous, warm, or tender. He has 3+ pretibial edema. The physical examination is otherwise normal.

1. Nephrotic syndrome is characterized by:
   A. Edema, hypoalbuminemia, and hypercholesterolemia
   B. Hypertension
   C. Proteinuria
   D. A and C
   E. All of the above

2. Possible complications of nephrotic syndrome include:
   A. Pneumococcal pneumonia and cellulitis
   B. Spontaneous bacterial peritonitis
   C. Pulmonary embolus
   D. Fatal cardiac arrhythmias
   E. A, B, and C

3. The initial treatment of uncomplicated childhood nephrotic syndrome is with:
   A. Corticosteroids
   B. Cyclophosphamide
   C. Cyclosporine
   D. Azathioprine
   E. Lovastatin

4. The most common cause of childhood nephrotic syndrome is:
   A. Post-streptococcal glomerulonephritis
   B. Membranous nephropathy
   C. Minimal change disease
   D. IgA nephropathy
   E. Focal segmental glomerulosclerosis

COMMENT

Pathophysiology • Nephrotic syndrome is characterized by proteinuria, hypoalbuminemia, edema, and hyperlipidemia. Urine protein loss is largely comprised of albumin and results from increased permeability of the glomerular capillary wall, the etiology of which is uncertain. Edema develops as a consequence of the resultant hypoalbuminemia and lowered oncotic pressure, usually first appearing when the serum albumin level is less than 2.5 g/dl. Hyperlipidemia is also a result of hypoproteinemia, through generalized increased protein synthesis in the liver and decreased lipid catabolism secondary to decreased plasma lipoprotein lipase, the major enzyme that removes lipids from the plasma.

Characteristics and etiology • Nephrotic syndrome is more common in boys than girls and it usually occurs between 2 and 6 years of age. Minimal change disease accounts for approximately 85% of all childhood nephrotic syndrome and is notable for its excellent response to steroids. Focal segmental glomerulosclerosis and membranous nephropathy are less frequent causes. Post-streptococcal renal disease is also a disease of childhood, however, as a cause of glomerulonephritis and not nephrotic syndrome.

Complications • The two major complications of nephrotic syndrome are infection and thrombosis, both secondary to urine loss of essential serum proteins. Factors increasing the risk of infection include decreased levels of immunoglobulin and opsonins as well as the mechanical effect of edema. The infections are predominantly caused by encapsulated organisms and include pneumonia, cellulitis, peritonitis, and sepsis. The increased risk of thrombosis is the result of decreased plasma levels of antithrombin III and, less often, proteins C and S, hyperaggregable platelets, and increased intravascular volume contraction.

Treatment • Supportive care of nephrotic syndrome includes efforts to minimize edema and avoid infection, including penicillin prophylaxis and pneumococcal vaccination, as well as salt restriction, intravenous albumin, and diuretic therapy. Therapy with immunomodulators specifically treats the illness. Fortunately, the most common cause of nephrotic syndrome in children, minimal change disease, responds well to corticosteroid therapy in more than 95% of cases. Only 20% of children with focal segmental glomerulosclerosis respond to corticosteroid and cytotoxic therapy, and it often progresses to end-stage renal disease.

Answers • 1-D 2-E 3-A 4-C

CASE PRESENTATION

A 9-year-old boy is brought to the emergency room after a load of building materials fell on him at a construction site. He is alert and oriented but has sustained a severe crush injury to his lower extremities. Immediate attention is paid to his orthopedic injuries. His creatinine kinase is 7000 U/L.

1. He is at risk for developing which one of the following?
   A. Syndrome of inappropriate antidiuretic hormone
   B. Myocardial infarction
   C. Transverse myelitis
   D. Rhabdomyolysis
   E. Pseudotumor cerebri

2. An indwelling bladder catheter is placed in the operating room and his urine is noted to be dark orange. The most likely cause is:
   A. Bleeding from catheterization
   B. Bilirubin in the urine
   C. Anesthestic complication
   D. Myoglobinuria
   E. Hemoglobinuria

3. Acceptable supportive care includes:
   A. Dialysis
   B. Plasmapheresis
   C. Urine alkalinization and correction of electrolyte abnormalities
   D. A and C
   E. All of the above

4. On the way back from the operating room he developed painful muscle spasms of his hands with flexion of his wrists and extension of his fingers. The most likely diagnosis is:
   A. Hypocalcemia
   B. Hypokalemia
   C. Anesthetic reaction
   D. Hyponatremia
   E. Acidosis

COMMENT

Rhabdomyolysis • Rhabdomyolysis occurs when striated muscle breaks down and releases cell constituents into the extracellular fluid and the circulation. One of the key compounds released is myoglobin. When massive amounts of myoglobin reach the renal urinary tract, it can cause a color change, obstruction, and renal dysfunction. The severity of rhabdomyolysis can vary from a subclinical rise of creatine kinase (CK) to a medical emergency including interstitial and muscle cell edema, contraction of intravascular volume, and pigment-induced acute renal failure (ARF). Today rhabdomyolysis is one of the leading causes of ARF. Therapy includes treatment of the underlying disorder, alkalinization of the urine with intravenous sodium bicarbonate to maintain the urine pH greater than 7, careful fluid and electrolyte management, and dialysis. Dialysis would be indicated for a rapidly rising serum creatinine level, volume overload, acidosis, electrolyte abnormality not responsive to medical management, and uremia with central nervous system changes. Life-threatening complications include hyperkalemia, severe acidosis, hypocalcemia, and hyperphosphatemia.

The patient is this case developed hypocalcemic tetany. Immediate therapy includes intravenous calcium replacement. Correction of low calcium levels is extremely difficult in the presence of low magnesium levels.

Answers • 1-D   2-D   3-D   4-A

JOINT PAIN IN AN ADOLESCENT

CASE PRESENTATION

A 16-year-old previously healthy female presents with a one month history of joint pain. She was on the school basketball team but has not been able to participate over the last two weeks secondary to her complaints. The joint pain waxes and wanes. It primarily involves her ankles and knees bilaterally and her left hand. Her review of systems is positive for decreased appetite and increasing fatigue. She is not on any medications. She does have a cousin who is on methotrexate for juvenile rheumatoid arthritis. On physical examination she is afebrile and her vital signs are within normal limits. She is thin appearing and muscular, in no acute distress. Her joint examination is normal but her skin examination is positive for a macular erythematous rash on her face involving her cheeks bilaterally and extending across her nasal bridge. The remainder of her physical exam is unremarkable. Initial laboratory evaluation reveals a normal basic metabolic panel and complete blood count. Liver function tests are within normal limits. An erythrocyte sedimentation rate is elevated.

1. Which of the following test results are consistent with the diagnosis of systemic lupus erythematosis (SLE)?
   A. Positive antinuclear antibody (ANA) in the homogenous pattern
   B. Positive anti-Smith antibody
   C. Positive anti-double-stranded DNA antibody
   D. Positive antineutrophil cytoplasmic antibody (ANCA)
   E. A, B, and C

2. The complications of lupus include:
   A. Nephritis
   B. Gallstones
   C. Pulmonary hypertension
   D. A and C
   E. A, B, and C

3. Further laboratory evaluation reveals a prolonged PTT, negative lupus anticoagulant, and positive VDRL. Which of the following statements are true?
   A. This patient is at risk for bleeding and should be treated with fresh frozen plasma prior to any surgical procedures.
   B. This patient has syphilis in addition to lupus and should be treated with a course of penicillin.
   C. This patient is at risk for thrombosis and should be tested for anticardiolipin or antiphospholipid antibody.
   D. These findings are likely secondary to lab error and no further evaluation or precautions are necessary.

4. The patient is treated with corticosteroids and plaquenil and responds well but then discontinues her treatment over the next two years. She then presents to an obstetrician, pregnant at 32 weeks gestation and with active SLE. Her newborn infant will be at increased risk for which of the following?
   A. Heart block
   B. Aseptic necrosis
   C. Hypoglycemia
   D. Lupus
   E. Congenital leukemia

COMMENT

Systemic lupus erythematosus (SLE) • SLE is a systemic disease of unknown etiology characterized by autoantibodies directed toward self-antigens that result in inflammatory damage to target organs. In a patient with active SLE, total hemolytic complement (CH50), C3, and C4 are all decreased. Antinuclear antibodies are easily measured and are often used as a screening tool for SLE. They are also positive in drug-induced lupus (i.e., from hydralazine), scleroderma, juvenile arthritis, juvenile dermatomyositis, and chronic active hepatitis. Levels of antibody to double-stranded DNA are more specific and reflect disease activity. Anti-Smith antibodies are only found in SLE, but do not reflect disease activity.

Characteristics • Patients present with a wide range of symptoms and signs including fatigue, prolonged fever, lymphadenopathy, arthralgias, arthritis, malar "butterfly" rash, discoid rash, pericarditis, seizures, transverse myelitis, nephritis, anemia, thrombocytopenia, neutropenia, psychiatric manifestations, and pulmonary hypertension or hemorrhage. Infants of mothers with active SLE are at risk for congenital heart block. In active SLE the PTT can be prolonged. This can be secondary to antibody against coagulation factors or lupus anticoagulant. Patients can also have a coexisting antiphospholipid syndrome with hypercoagulability and risk of thrombosis. These patients may have an antiphospholipid antibody, anticardiolipin antibody, or a false-positive VDRL.

Treatment • Treatment of SLE is varied based on the manifestations and severity of the disease. Treatment includes symptomatic treatment of the arthralgias with non-steroidal anti-inflammatory agents. Moderate to severe forms are initially treated with corticosteroids. Other agents commonly used include plaquenil, mycophenolate mofetil, and azathioprine. Treatment with intravenous cyclophosphamide is reserved for treatment of severe forms of the disease.

Answers • 1-E 2-D 3-C 4-A

CASE PRESENTATION

A 2-year-old boy presents with slowly progressive hoarseness of his voice and inspiratory stridor. There is no history of fever or other symptoms. He was born at full term gestation with no complications. Prenatal history is significant for a maternal history of genital lesions, removed surgically several years before. Maternal prenatal laboratory tests were normal. On physical examination, the patient has a hoarse voice but breathes comfortably, with stridor when upset and crying.

From the options below, select the appropriate choice for questions 1-6:
- A. Laryngeal web
- B. Larynotracheomalacia
- C. Laryngotracheobronchitis
- D. Foreign body
- E. Laryngeal papilloma
- F. Respiratory hemangioma

For a patient with inspiratory stridor with each of the following clinical descriptions, select the most likely diagnosis:

1. Rapid growth in the first 2 months of life
2. Inspiratory stridor at birth, worsened in supine position, that gradually resolves by about 18 months of age
3. Weak cry and stridor present at birth
4. Acute onset of barking cough and inspiratory stridor
5. Acute onset of cough followed by stridor
6. Maternal genital warts

In the patient described above, a chest radiograph reveals no obvious abnormalities. Lateral radiograph of the neck reveals a possible pedunculated mass.

7. What is the most likely etiologic agent of the mass?
   - A. *Haemophilus influenzae* type B
   - B. Human herpes virus 6
   - C. Human papilloma virus
   - D. Parvovirus
   - E. *Treponema pallidum*

8. What were the lesions that the mother had several years ago?
   - A. Chancroid
   - B. Condyloma acuminata
   - C. Melanoma
   - D. Primary syphilis
   - E. Genital herpes

COMMENT

Stridor • Respiratory obstruction outside of the thorax results in stridor, the sound generated as air is pulled past the airway narrowing during inspiration. Clinical conditions that result in stridor and features of each include: (1) laryngeal webs—a congenital anomaly usually also affecting the vocal cords such that the infant has a weak cry, (2) laryngotracheomalacia—a relative laxity of the laryngeal and tracheal cartilage that gradually improves with age, (3) laryngotracheobronchitis or croup—an infection, usually viral, commonly affecting preschool children with sudden onset of a "barking" cough and respiratory distress that worsens each night for several days, (4) aspirated foreign body—the bane of toddlers who put every object in their mouths, usually presenting with acute onset of a cough in an otherwise well child that may then develop stridor and distress as edema and obstruction becomes more severe, (5) laryngeal hemangioma—infants often have rapidly enlarging hemangiomas that are usually of no consequence but if they occur in the respiratory tract may cause obstruction, and (6) respiratory papilloma—caused by human papilloma virus infection, causing laryngeal lesions or lesions throughout the respiratory tract.

Human papillomavirus (HPV) • HPV infections can manifest in many ways, depending on the area of the body involved. The lesions are usually due to hyperkeratotic changes in the skin layers. Laryngeal papillomatosis is one such manifestation, most commonly caused by HPV types 6 and 11, with exposure during birth. HPV is usually spread by direct contact. The lesions that occur in childhood may be due to contact with vaginal or genital lesions during birth, although even children born by cesarean section may develop laryngeal papillomas. Family history is positive for HPV infection in 50% of cases of the childhood onset laryngeal papillomas. The laryngeal lesions that occur later in life may be due to exposure through sexual activity. Diagnosis is best made via direct visualization by laryngoscope. Radiographic studies are usually indicated in children with new onset of stridor or wheezing and may help in diagnosing this lesion as well. The differential diagnosis includes any obstructive lesion of the larynx and vocal cords.

Treatment • Lesions may regress spontaneously or may worsen without treatment. Treatment is difficult and often involves endoscopic surgery and treatment with various cytotoxic or cytoinhibitory agents. The disease may progress and result in intrapulmonary spread of the disease, resulting in cystic and ultimately restrictive lung disease.

Answers • 1-F 2-B 3-A 4-C 5-D 6-E 7-C 8-B

CASE PRESENTATION

A 9-month-old Caucasian girl is brought into her primary pediatrician's office with a four-day history of recurrent fevers as high as 104 degrees rectally. The child was seen in an emergency department two days before where she was diagnosed with acute otitis media and started on amoxicillin. At that examination the emergency department physician noted that the child's pharynx was erythematous. Since that emergency department evaluation, the patient has been sleepy, irritable, and has not eaten well, with increased spitting up and loose stools.

From the options below, select the appropriate choice for questions 1-5:

A. Meningitis
B. Acute otitis media not responding to the antibiotic
C. Dehydration
D. Febrile seizure
E. Intussusception

For this patient and the additional history or physical examination finding listed below, select the most likely diagnosis.

1. History of jerking movement of arms and legs for five minutes followed by lethargy
2. Crying with flexion of neck
3. Flexing legs and crying
4. Decreased frequency of wet diapers
5. Bulging tympanic membranes

Additional history reveals that the fever resolved the night before and since that time, a rash developed, initially on the patient's trunk and has spread diffusely. On physical examination, the patient does indeed have a rash, greatest on the trunk but to a lesser extent on the extremities and face, consisting of pink macules with a subtle white halo surrounding the lesions.

6. The most likely etiology of this child's illness is:

A. Human herpes virus 6
B. Drug reaction
C. Epstein-Barr virus
D. Parvovirus B19
E. *Streptococcus pyogenes* group A

7. This disease is known as:

A. Fifth disease
B. Erythema infectiosum
C. Erythema toxicum
D. Roseola infantum
E. Scarlet fever

COMMENT

Infants with fever • The differential diagnosis of fever in infants and young children is extensive and the full spectrum of illness must be carefully considered in each case as children have limited presentations and often appear relatively well until they are close to cardiovascular collapse. Meningitis and sepsis must always be part of the differential, especially as infants cannot complain of headache and usually do not develop papilledema. The anterior fontanel can be used as a pressure gauge for estimating intracranial pressure in a young infant, as it is often bulging in cases of meningitis and other causes of increased intracranial pressure, but in older infants as the anterior fontanel becomes smaller and more fibrous, this finding is unreliable. Children with fever from any etiology should also be carefully examined for dehydration and their symptomatic care should include adequate fluids for the increased losses with fever. High fevers, especially when the rise in temperature is very sudden, may cause febrile seizures, usually occurring in children between the ages of 9 months and 5 years.

Roseola infantum • Roseola, also known as exanthema subitum, is the sixth in a series of historically described erythematous rashes in children: first disease (measles), second disease (rubella), third disease (scarlet fever), fourth disease (Duke's disease or scarlatiniform rash), and fifth disease (erythema infectiosum or parvovirus B19). It is now known to be caused by human herpes virus 6. Diagnosis of this disease is very difficult prior to the onset of the rash, as the symptoms are nonspecific and include high fever, pharyngitis, erythematous tympanic membranes, lymphadenopathy, gastrointestinal complaints, and irritability. The classic rash occurs coincident with defervescence on the third or fourth day of illness and usually lasts three to four days. The peak incidence of this disease is between 6 months and 3 years of age.

Complications • Roseola is generally self-limited and benign, requiring only symptomatic care such as adequate hydration. Because of the high fever and the age at which roseola occurs, febrile seizures have been seen in a significant number of children during this illness. It may rarely be associated with intussusception, with intestinal lymphadenopathy as a lead point.

Answers • 1-D 2-A 3-E 4-C 5-B 6-A 7-D

Section 2

Psychiatry

Michael A. de Arellano, PhD
Mary C. Fields, MD
Patricia L. Fiero, PhD
D. Walter Hiott, MD
Matthew S. Koval, MD
Jerome E. Kurent, MD, MPH
Himanshu P. Upadhyaya, MBBS, MS
Jessica A. Whiteley, PhD

BEHAVIORAL DISTURBANCE OF CHILDHOOD

CASE PRESENTATION

A 9-year-old African-American male presents to his primary care physician with a three-week history of problematic changes in his behaviors in both the school and home settings. His teachers report that the child has been inattentive and increasingly argumentative since returning from a one-week school break. The mother reports her son is more irritable than usual and has difficulty falling asleep. She also notes that he has recently begun slapping and punching his siblings. The youth reports that his "belly hurts" and he denies feeling sad or crying. There is no past medical history of gastrointestinal problems and no recent change of bowel, bladder, or appetite. Vital signs are stable and normal. Physical exam of the abdomen is without findings.

1. At this point, the physician should be most concerned about assessing the youth for:
   A. Thoughts of violence to himself or acts of self-harm or injury
   B. Access to firearms in the home or community
   C. Thoughts of physical violence against others
   D. All of the above
   E. A and B only

2. In adolescents and children, the only FDA-approved antidepressant for the treatment of childhood or adolescent depression is:
   A. Bupropion
   B. Sertraline
   C. Fluoxetine
   D. Citalopram
   E. None of the above

3. A reasonable medication and starting dose to prescribe for the symptoms found in this 9-year-old male is:
   A. Methylphenidate 20 mg by mouth twice a day
   B. Citalopram 40 mg by mouth every morning
   C. Sertraline 50 mg by mouth every morning
   D. Venlafaxine 150 mg by mouth three times a day
   E. Fluoxetine 40 mg every day

COMMENT

Risk assessment • Inattentiveness, difficulty falling asleep, recent changes of behaviors, and irritability are all symptoms of depression in children and adolescents. In this population disruption of behavior often presents as the main symptom of depression. Children are more likely to report "I'm not good" or "I wish I had never been born" rather than endorsing a sad mood or crying. In any depressed or behaviorally disturbed person, suicidal or homicidal ideation must be assessed. Access to firearms increases the likelihood of completion of suicide or homicide. When access to firearms is known to be present, families, friends, or authorities should remove the firearm(s) from that environment to reduce the risk of harm to self and/or others. Physicians should remind adults that a "hidden" gun in the home or telling kids not to "touch" or "play with" the gun are inadequate precautions for the often impulsive and inquisitive young. The most reliable source for assessing suicidal thoughts in a child or teen is to ASK the child or teen. It is not uncommon for young persons to "protect" their parents from such morbid or frightening thoughts by not telling them. Additionally, the physician needs to speak directly to the parents as they may have seen, have discovered, or know something that the young person does not endorse, and they most certainly need to know if their child or teen is suicidal.

Pediatric indications • As of 2002, no antidepressant has been approved for the treatment of childhood or adolescent depression. Fluvoxamine (Luvox) and Sertraline (Zoloft) have been approved for obsessive-compulsive disorders of childhood while imipramine is approved for enuresis. Medications commonly used in the treatment of pediatric disorders or illnesses, including antibiotics, have been insufficiently studied in the young to receive FDA approval for pediatric use.

Reasonable medication • Sertraline (Zoloft) is an SSRI that may be safely started at a low dose of either 25 or 50 mg by mouth every day. The optimal therapeutic response may be achieved at a higher dose and should be adjusted based upon clinical response of the child. Still, at the optimal dose for that child, the maximal benefit may not occur until after a four- to eight-week treatment period has passed. Starting any antidepressant at the higher end of the dosing recommendations is likely to cause more side effects than benefits early in the treatment. Methylphenidate is rarely used in pediatric care of depression, although it is commonly used to control ADHD symptoms. Venlafaxine is less commonly used in children or teens than the SSRIs as it is even less studied in this population than the SSRIs are. Also, the 150 mg three times a day dosing is an aggressive starting dose for an adult, much less a child.

Answers • 1-D 2-E 3-C

ATTENTION DEFICIT/HYPERACTIVITY DISORDER

● CASE PRESENTATION

A 5-year-old Caucasian male presents with his mother to your office for evaluation of behavior problems. The mother reports that she worries her son may be brain damaged ever since he was hit in the head by a baseball at age 2. She tells you that at the time of injury her son was evaluated in the ER but "they didn't find anything but a big old knot on his head." She recalls that her son did not lose consciousness with the trauma. Nonetheless, she reports that ever since he was 3 years old he "can't sit still," seems to always be "wound up," and has difficulty falling asleep. She further reports that "even at church they asked me to have him seen by a doctor" because he cannot sit still during Sunday school like the other children. She goes on to say, "he can sit still for hours playing his computer games. Doctor, help me! I'm worn out!" While you are speaking with the mother, you cannot help but notice how tired you are becoming as you, your nurse, and his mother keep redirecting the boy out of the many drawers and cabinets full of medical supplies. When you speak directly to the child he often looks out the window or into the hallway and says "huh?" to many of your questions.

1. The diagnosis of ADHD requires at least six symptoms of attention problems and/or hyperactivity and impulsivity plus:
   A. Symptoms must cause impairment in at least two different settings
   B. Maladaptive behaviors that are inconsistent with developmental age
   C. Impairment in social, occupational, or academic functioning
   D. A predominantly inattentive, predominantly hyperkinetic and impulsive, or a combination of these types of symptoms
   E. All of the above

2. In order to diagnose ADHD the symptoms must have been present for at least:
   A. Six days
   B. Six weeks
   C. Six months
   D. One year
   E. Any period of time as long as the symptoms cause impairment

3. If a physician can do only ONE thing to help an ADHD child it should be:
   A. Refer the child for behavioral therapy
   B. Recommend a low-sugar, low-caffeine diet
   C. Refer the child for social skills group therapy
   D. Parent education on how to parent energetic children
   E. Prescribe a psychostimulant

● COMMENT

Diagnostic criteria • All of the features listed are a part of the ADHD diagnosis. ADHD may be subtyped as described based upon symptom clusters. Hyperactive symptoms are fidgeting, squirming in seat, running about or climbing excessively in situations not suuitable for such behaviors, speaking loudly in activities, often being "on the go," and talking excessively. Impulsive symptoms include blurting out answers before questions are completed, difficulty waiting turn, often interrupting others, or intruding upon others. Inattentive symptoms consist of failing to pay close attention to details or making careless mistakes, often seeming to not listen, difficulty maintaining attention to tasks or play activities, often unable to complete chores, assignments or duties, or failing to finish school assignments and often losing things like school assignments, pencils, papers, or toys. Six or more symptoms must be present from any of these categories to diagnose ADHD.

Duration • According to the DSM-IV TR criteria, the symptoms of ADHD must have been present for at least six months. ADHD may be diagnosed at any age but the onset of symptoms must predate age 7. Today, most children with ADHD are not diagnosed or are not receiving treatment for their condition. Conversely some children may be inappropriately diagnosed with ADHD when they actually may suffer from a learning disability or developmental delays.

First but not only • More than any other intervention, psychostimulants are the best choice of intervention to reduce symptoms and the adverse sequelae of untreated ADHD. Specifically, psychostimulants allow increased academic and social performance and reduce risk for substance abuse and early sexual experiences, lowering teen pregnancy and incarceration rates in the medication-treated groups as compared to behavior or other modes of therapy.

Answers • 1-E 2-C 3-E

CASE PRESENTATION

A 13-year-old Hispanic female presents with her parents to your office for assessment of an ever-worsening problem with "not eating" and weight loss. According to the parents, the daughter was a normal healthy and active adolescent until about eight months ago. About that time, the daughter had taken a cruise to the Bahamas with her school theater group. Upon her return from that trip, the parents noticed a gradual reduction of her meal intake so that now she only eats one small bowl of lettuce and tomatoes once a day. At first, the parents report they were not concerned, but now the daughter's weight loss scares them. The daughter smiles often and answers all your questions with "everything is fine" and "I don't have a problem." Her height is 5'7" tall and she weighs 102 lbs. wearing only a hospital gown.

1. The MOST important lab test to get in the initial evaluation of an anorexic patient is:
   A. Serum cortisol level
   B. Basic metabolic panel (Chem 7)
   C. AST and ALT
   D. Serum albumin and prealbumin levels
   E. Estrogen, testosterone, LH, and FSH levels

2. Anorexia nervosa remains one of the most lethal of psychiatric disorders. Having a mortality of 5.6% per decade of illness, the proximal cause of death in anorexic patients is most commonly:
   A. Cardiac arrhythmias leading to cardiac arrest
   B. Global hypometabolism of the CNS
   C. Hypovolemic nephropathy
   D. Starvation
   E. Pulmonary edema

3. Caution must be exercised when first beginning the refeeding or nutritional rehabilitation stage of AN treatment because:
   A. Fluid overload can occur and may lead to pulmonary edema
   B. GI dysmotility can cause obstruction in overly aggressive refeeding
   C. Renal function and liver function may be compromised
   D. Extreme and painful bloating of the abdominal cavity and bowel changes or even the resumption of bowel movements may be a slow and complicated course
   E. All of the above

COMMENT

Laboratory data • The most important lab study to get is a basic metabolic panel or Chem 7. It is imperative to assess the status of electrolytes, particularly sodium, potassium, and chloride serum levels, and renal functioning as suggested by the blood urea nitrogen (BUN) and creatinine levels. Also, the glycemic state can be assessed. All of these may help the physician avert any acute medical crisis such as cardiac arrhythmias due to electrolyte imbalances or acute renal failure associated with dehydration and malnutrition state. Serum calcium levels are also important as this ion directly impacts cardiac functioning. All other labs listed are helpful in assessing the full impact the malnourished state has on the body but are less urgent in the initial work-up. Albumin and prealbumin levels may reflect the severity and, to a lesser extent, the duration of the starvation state. AST and ALT will aid in assessing the liver function; knowing the total protein and direct and indirect bilirubin levels would also be informative. By definition, an anorexic female would not be having menses, thus an elevated FSH is expected with low estrogen (associated with lanugo).

Mortality • Cardiac arrhythmias are the most proximal cause of death in an anorexic patient. This is a direct result of severe electrolyte imbalances and poor cardiac muscle functioning in a starved state. Serum cortisol may be elevated and reveal the stressed state of the malnourished body. In a restricting-only anorexia patient, there is no expectation of finding specific oral cavity problems as would be expected in either a binge-eating/purging type of anorexia nervosa patient or a purging bulimia nervosa patient. Similarly, there would be no specific oral cavity finding in a nonpurging bulimia nervosa patient.

Complications • All of these adverse outcomes are possible in the refeeding stage of treatment. Thus, overly aggressive refeeding may do more harm and is to be avoided.

Answers • 1-B 2-A 3-E

CASE PRESENTATION

Denise is a 7-year-old girl who was referred to you to assess and treat behavior problems that developed two years ago shortly after having been sexually abused by her 16-year-old male cousin. Her parents report being very concerned because she is acting out at home, is persistently oppositional and noncompliant with their instructions, and is having significant difficulty at school. Of particular concern to her parents is their child's sexual acting-out behavior. They report that she has been masturbating in public, both through her clothing and under her clothing. They note that she engages in this behavior at home, but not at school. The patient's mother reports getting very upset when she finds her child engaging in this behavior. She is concerned that her child may sexually abuse another child when she grows up. There are no other children in their home.

1. How common is child sexual abuse among women?
   A. Less than 1%
   B. 5% to 10%
   C. 15% to 30%
   D. 45% to 60%
   E. Over 80%

2. Based on the information presented above, what is the most likely diagnosis?
   A. PTSD
   B. ADHD
   C. Adjustment disorder with disturbance of conduct
   D. Acute stress disorder
   E. Reactive attachment disorder

3. What treatment intervention has had the most empirical support of treating behaviors such as public masturbation in this case?
   A. Help the child to gain insight into why she is doing this
   B. Nondirective play therapy
   C. Behavior therapy focused on reducing the behavior as you would treat other inappropriate behaviors
   D. Aversive therapy
   E. Aquatic therapy

4. The patient's mother expresses concern that her child may grow up to perpetrate sexual abuse. How likely is it that this will occur?
   A. 95% chance
   B. 75% chance
   C. 50% chance
   D. 25% chance
   E. Less than 10% chance

COMMENT

Prevalence • Current estimates of the prevalence of sexual abuse vary depending on study methodology (e.g., definitions of sexual abuse, sampling differences). Prevalence estimates in nationally representative samples have reported the risks of about 1 in 8 to 1 in 3 in women, with the majority occurring prior to 18 years of age. Estimates for men are lower and more variable.

Diagnosis • Based on this presentation, the most likely diagnosis is adjustment disorder with disturbance of conduct. The symptoms developed shortly after an identified stressor (Criterion A). She is experiencing impairment at school and at home (Criterion B). Criteria for another diagnosis is not fully met (Criterion C), and the symptoms would not be considered bereavement. Because the symptoms have continued beyond six months (Criterion E), the diagnosis would be specified as "chronic."

Treatment • Behavioral interventions have been used effectively to reduce public masturbation and similar inappropriate behaviors. It would be important to gain a better understanding of the precipitants and consequences to the behavior. Often these behaviors are very upsetting to parents, who may respond in a strong emotional manner, and possibly inadvertently reinforce the behavior. Parents should be provided information on the commonness of such behaviors and on how to treat these behaviors as you would other inappropriate behaviors.

Perpetration risk • A common myth about sexually abused children is that most of them grow up to be perpetrators of sexual abuse themselves. Earlier research in this area focused on whether perpetrators of sexual abuse were themselves sexually abused, rather than whether a community sample of individuals sexually abused as children engage in the perpetration of sexual abuse. The former strategy, which tended to use prison or clinical populations of sexual abuse perpetrators, overestimated the prevalence. More recent estimates place the prevalence of such behaviors below 5%. Nonetheless, precautions (e.g., increased supervision, safety planning) should be taken when other children are in the home with a child who has experienced sexual abuse.

Answers • 1-C 2-C 3-C 4-E

DEVELOPMENTAL, GENDER, AND CULTURAL CONSIDERATIONS IN MAJOR DEPRESSIVE DISORDER IN CHILDREN

● CASE PRESENTATION

Ernesto is an 11-year-old, Mexican-American boy who was referred for assessment and treatment of behavior problems at home and at school. His mother reports that he seems very sensitive and is easily "set off." She describes several incidents in which he has gotten into arguments over minor things, often getting very frustrated and crying. She notes that he has not been getting along well with his siblings or friends in the neighborhood, and no longer is interested in school activities in which he previously participated. Instead, he prefers to spend time in his room surfing the Internet. At school, his teacher reports that he has difficulty concentrating, and she notes that he does not engage other children much and sits alone during lunch. Ernesto's mother is also concerned because he has missed numerous days of school because of headaches and stomachaches, he has not been eating as well, and he has been sleeping a lot more than usual. Ernesto denied any depressed mood, and says that he is "fine" and just wants to be left alone.

1. What is the most likely diagnosis?
   A. Major depressive disorder
   B. Generalized anxiety disorder
   C. Attention deficit hyperactivity disorder
   D. Posttraumatic stress disorder
   E. Oppositional defiant disorder

2. In recent years, the diagnostic criteria for depression in adults has been modified for children and adolescents to include _____, which can be used to substitute for depressed mood?
   A. Insomnia
   B. Attention problems
   C. Irritable mood
   D. Mania
   E. Crying spells

3. When assessing for depression in younger children and in children or adults from some ethnic minority groups (e.g., Hispanic, Asian), it is particularly important to also do a thorough assessment of which of the following types of symptoms, which have a greater likelihood of co-occurring with depression and anxiety symptoms in these groups?
   A. Neurocognitive
   B. Somatic
   C. Manic
   D. Dissociative
   E. Psychotic

4. Although women are about twice as likely as men to be depressed, in younger children:
   A. The rates are about equal
   B. Boys are five times more likely to be depressed than girls
   C. Girls are five times more likely to be depressed than boys
   D. Boys are twice as likely as girls to be depressed
   E. Girls are ten times as likely as boys to be depressed

● COMMENT

Diagnostic criteria • Ernesto meets five of the nine Criterion A symptoms for a major depressive disorder. These include diminished interest in activities, decrease in appetite, insomnia, diminished ability to concentrate, and irritable mood (see age-related differences). Although there may be some overlap with each of the other listed diagnoses, the MDD diagnosis appears most appropriate.

Age-related differences • Although depressed affect does not seem to be a predominant symptom, significant irritability has been reported and can be used as a substitute for depressed mood when applying DSM-IV criteria to children and adolescents. This substitution reflects research and clinical findings that children and adolescents often exhibit irritability when depressed.

Ethnic differences • An additional developmental issue that should be considered when working with children is that research has found younger children to have a greater tendency to report somatic complaints when depressed. This phenomenon tends to diminish in adolescence and adulthood. Similarly, children and adults from some ethnic minority groups (e.g., Hispanic, Asian) have also been found to report more somatic symptoms with the occurrence of depressive or anxiety symptoms.

Gender differences in childhood • Developmental changes appear to exist in the prevalence of depression across sexes. That is, among children rates of depression appear to be similar for boys and girls; however, the rates for adult women double those of adult men. At what point in development this change in prevalence occurs and why these differences exist remains unclear and requires further investigation.

Answers • 1-A   2-C   3-B   4-A

CASE PRESENTATION

Susan is a 22-year-old female who is a senior at a local university. She presents with significant distress secondary to a sexual assault by an acquaintance that occurred six months ago. Her symptoms include having intrusive thoughts, images, and nightmares about the assault; feelings of numbness; feeling jumpy and startling easily; and having difficulty sleeping. She also reports significant distress in and avoidance of many situations and places, including parking garages and enclosed spaces (e.g., elevators). Similarly, she has been avoiding going out with her friends to bars, and is particularly distressed if she finds herself in a situation where she is alone with a man (e.g., arrives to class early and the only other individual there is a male student). In addition, she also reports feeling nauseated when she smells strong cologne or beer, or hears loud music. You also learn that she is having great difficulty engaging in sexual activities with her current boyfriend, and even becomes distressed if they kiss for extended periods of time. After further assessment of the sexual assault, you learn that she was assaulted by a male acquaintance who had agreed to drive her home after they met for drinks at a bar. Once in the car, which was parked in the college garage, he sexually assaulted her. She reports that during the assault she persistently feared that he was going to hurt her. She feels hopeless and says she does not feel she will ever get better. She particularly remembers how loud the music seemed, the strong smell of his cologne and beer on his breath, and persistently fearing that he was going to seriously hurt her.

1. Given this information, what is Susan's most likely diagnosis?
   A. Major depressive disorder
   B. Adjustment disorder
   C. Acute stress disorder
   D. Posttraumatic stress disorder (PTSD)
   E. Obsessive-compulsive disorder

2. Which of the following is relevant to a differential diagnosis of PTSD versus acute stress disorder?
   A. Length of time since traumatic event
   B. Presence of depressive symptoms
   C. Symptoms persisting for more than one month
   D. Symptoms were present prior to the trauma
   E. Severity of symptoms

3. What treatment intervention is recommended to address psychological distress or physiological reactivity to trauma-related cues and/or avoidance of such cues?
   A. Relaxation therapy
   B. Biofeedback
   C. Response prevention
   D. Exposure therapy
   E. Medication trial

4. Flooding, systematic desensitization, and implosion are all methods of what type of treatment intervention?
   A. Relaxation therapy
   B. Biofeedback
   C. Response prevention
   D. Exposure therapy
   E. Cognitive therapy

COMMENT

Diagnosis • Based on this information, the most likely diagnosis would be PTSD. The patient meets DSM-IV Criterion A: having experienced a traumatic event in which she perceived threat of death or serious injury and in which she responded with intense fear; Criterion B: re-experiencing of the event (e.g., nightmares, intrusive thoughts, distress in response to reminders); Criterion C: persistent avoidance of reminders and emotional numbing (e.g., avoiding parking garages and bars, feeling numb); and Criterion D: persistent increased arousal (difficulty sleeping, feeling jumpy, possible hypervigilance). Finally, the patient also reports clinically significant distress and social impairment (Criterion F).

Duration of symptoms • In addition, the patient reports duration of symptoms of more than one month (Criterion E); this would also distinguish it from acute stress disorder, in which symptoms can only last four weeks.

Treatment of choice • The intervention of choice to treat distress associated with trauma-related cues is exposure. This intervention is thought to help break the conditioned association between the trauma-related cue and the patient's fear response. Exposure can be presented in vivo or imaginally. Although two medications (sertraline and paroxetine) currently are FDA-approved for use in treating PTSD, this should be considered adjunctive therapy to the psychotherapy. A treatment plan for PTSD should never consist of pharmacotherapy alone.

Variations • Exposure-based interventions may also be provided in gradual (e.g., systematic desensitization) or intensive (e.g., flooding, implosion) formats. Such exposure-based treatment is also commonly used for the treatment of specific phobias.

Answers • 1-D 2-C 3-D 4-D

CASE PRESENTATION

A 7-year-old boy is seen with his parents with the chief complaint of a long history of "behavior problems." The parents report his second-grade school performance is not good, and he constantly requires redirection at home and school secondary to disruptive behavior and "fidgeting." He cries a lot, and is immature compared to his peers. After receiving a time-out for acting out at home recently, he commented that he wished he were dead.

1. Which of the following disorders should be in the differential diagnosis?
   A. Depressive disorder
   B. ADHD
   C. Anxiety disorder
   D. Learning disorder
   E. All of the above

2. After a complete evaluation, ADHD is diagnosed. The best treatment for the patient from the following list is:
   A. Mixed amphetamine salts 10 mg once per day
   B. Pemoline 75 mg each day
   C. Methylphenidate 5 to 10 mg at 7 a.m., 11 a.m., and 3 p.m.
   D. Imipramine 50 mg twice a day
   E. Behavioral modification and no medication

3. Common side effects of stimulant treatment include which of the following?
   A. Headache
   B. Stomach pain
   C. Poor appetite
   D. Agitation
   E. All of the above

4. Which of the following should be monitored frequently in patients taking stimulants?
   A. Weight
   B. Height
   C. Emergence of motor or vocal tics
   D. Pulse/BP
   E. All of the above

COMMENT

Differential diagnosis of problematic behavior • Although this patient's history is indicative of ADHD, one must always rule out other disorders that have the final common pathway of "behavior problems." Other disorders to consider would be adjustment disorders, hearing/vision problems, and oppositional defiant disorder. All of the disorders are not only part of the differential diagnosis of ADHD, but can also be found comorbidly in children with ADHD. A complete diagnostic evaluation and screening is essential in children with behavior problems.

Treatment of ADHD • The best initial treatment for ADHD, according to recent studies, is achieved through short-acting stimulants (methylphenidate, d-amphetamine, or amphetamine salts) on a three times a day schedule. This dosing regimen has been shown to be superior to behavior treatment alone, behavior treatment plus methylphenidate three times a day, and short-acting stimulants twice a day. Prescribing amphetamine salts once each morning is usually not adequate because the half-life, although slightly longer than methylphenidate, is still roughly only six hours and would not provide adequate coverage for a full day of school and homework. Pemoline is not considered first-line treatment for ADHD as there have been more than a dozen cases of liver failure associated with its use over the last 20 years. Imipramine has been shown to be helpful for ADHD, but again would not be considered first-line due to the associated side effects of prolongation of Q-T interval and the resulting dysrhythmia that may occur in rare individuals.

Side effects of stimulant therapy • The common side effects of stimulant medications are listed in question 3. Other side effects of stimulants include nervousness, insomnia, dizziness, and palpitations. Less common, but potentially serious effects include psychosis, arrhythmias, tic disorders, abuse, and dependency. Bradycardia is generally NOT seen with stimulants, and in fact tachycardia is a relatively common problem.

Monitoring patients on stimulants • In addition to monitoring for clinical effectiveness and improved behavior and academic performance, health care providers should monitor height, weight, and vital signs. Stimulants can sometimes exacerbate or uncover tic disorders in patients, so monitoring for tics in patients on stimulants is also important.

Answers • 1-E 2-C 3-E 4-E

CASE PRESENTATION

A 28-year-old woman with bipolar disorder has recently moved to the area and needs medication follow-up. She has been on lithium carbonate for four years and reports it works "fairly well." She reports that she has not had any laboratory studies performed in over a year. She currently lives with her boyfriend and quit using birth control pills several months ago because she feels they were causing weight gain.

1. Which of the following lists of lab tests are most appropriate to order for this patient?
   A. Basic metabolic panel, liver panel, beta-HCG
   B. Basic metabolic panel, thyroid panel, lithium level
   C. Basic metabolic panel, CBC, lithium level, beta-HCG
   D. Thyroid panel, lithium level, liver panel
   E. Basic metabolic panel, thyroid panel, lithium level, beta-HCG

2. The following lithium levels are appropriate for acute mania and chronic lithium prophylaxis:
   A. Acute: 1.4–1.9 mmol/L; Chronic: 0.6–0.8 mmol/L
   B. Acute: 1.0–1.2 mmol/L; Chronic: 0.1–0.4 mmol/L
   C. Acute: 1.0–1.2 mmol/L; Chronic: 0.6–1.0 mmol/L
   D. Acute: 0.8–1.0 mmol/L; Chronic: 0.8–1.0 mmol/L
   E. None of the above

3. Side effects associated with lithium therapy include which of the following?
   A. Weight gain
   B. Polydipsia
   C. Polyuria
   D. Sedation
   E. All of the above

4. The following medications have FDA approval for use in bipolar affective disorder:
   A. Lamotrigine
   B. Valproate
   C. Gabapentin
   D. Carbamazepine
   E. All of the above

COMMENT

Monitoring patients on lithium therapy • When a patient is on lithium therapy, it is important to follow electrolytes and BUN/creatinine with a basic metabolic panel. Thyroid function should be monitored because lithium can interfere with the production of thyroid hormone and may lead to hypothyroidism (which may cause depressive symptoms). All women of childbearing years should have beta-HCG checked, particularly when unprotected intercourse is occurring. Lithium is a known teratogenic agent (especially Ebstein's anomaly of the tricuspid valve) in a developing fetus. Finally, a lithium level should be periodically checked to assure compliance and a therapeutic level.

Lithium levels • When lithium is used prophylactically, levels should be between 0.6 and 1.0. Although some individuals can get by with lower levels (−0.4), it would be ill advised to go much lower than that. In acute mania, lithium levels generally need to be slightly higher, in the 1.0 to 1.2 range, but levels at 1.4 or greater are often associated with very problematic side effects and/or toxicity.

Side effects of lithium therapy • Common side effects of lithium use include GI complaints, tremor, sedation, lethargy, polyuria, polydipsia, and nocturia.

FDA approved medications for bipolar disorder • The only current FDA-approved medications for long-term mood stabilization in bipolar affective disorder are lithium and valproate. Olanzapine also has FDA approval for the treatment of short-term mania associated with bipolar disorder. The other medications listed have certainly been used for treatment of bipolar disorder with varying degrees of success, but at this point they are considered "off label."

Answers • 1-E 2-C 3-E 4-B

THE RELUCTANT SCHIZOPHRENIC

CASE PRESENTATION

A 22-year-old female with an 11-month history of schizophrenia, undifferentiated type, presents to the mental-health clinic for medication follow-up. Records indicate long-standing noncompliance with haloperidol and benztropine, the only medications prescribed thus far. The patient reports she will not take the "poison" that is causing her muscles to ache and stiffen. She and her parents request a new medication to treat her psychotic symptoms.

1. Which of the following medications would be an appropriate agent to switch the patient to?
   A. Fluphenazine
   B. Trifluoperazine
   C. Olanzapine
   D. Perphenazine
   E. Thiothixene

2. High-potency antipsychotics are more likely than low-potency agents to cause which of the following side effects?
   A. Sedation
   B. Anticholinergic side effects
   C. Extrapyramidal side effects
   D. Orthostatic hypotension
   E. Dry mouth

3. The following antipsychotics are currently available in "depot" form:
   A. Haloperidol
   B. Fluphenazine
   C. Quetiapine
   D. A and B
   E. A, B, and C

COMMENT

New medications with fewer side effects • Chronically mentally ill patients have a difficult time taking medications for several reasons. Many chronically psychotic patients have paranoid thoughts that cause them to be distrustful of treatment providers and medications. In addition, many psychiatric medications are beset with problematic side effects. When a patient is noncompliant with antipsychotic medication secondary to extrapyramidal side effects (EPS), one should consider using a newer so-called "atypical" antipsychotic. These newer drugs are much less likely to cause EPS and the problem of tardive dyskinesia (a chronic and sometimes irreversible movement disorder caused by neuroleptic medications). Atypical agents also have the benefit of improving positive and negative symptoms of schizophrenia, while more traditional medications seem to improve mostly positive symptoms. Positive symptoms include hallucinations and delusions while negative symptoms include social withdrawal, flat affect, and difficulty with decision making. Atypical antipsychotics include clozapine, risperidone, olanzapine, quetiapine, and ziprasidone. Most psychiatrists consider atypical agents to be the treatment of choice for chronic psychosis.

High vs. low potency antipsychotics • High potency antipsychotics are generally associated with high extrapyramidal side effects (EPS), but low sedation and anticholinergic effects. This would be the opposite of the low potency agents, which, in addition to causing orthostatic hypotension, have a high degree of sedation and anticholinergic side effects but low EPS. The atypical neuroleptics generally do not fit this "high potency vs. low potency paradigm, and must be looked at individually in terms of side-effect profile.

Depot neuroleptics • Using depot formulations of antipsychotic medication can improve compliance (unless the noncompliance is due to the particular side effects of high potency agents). The only two antipsychotics available in depot form are haloperidol and fluphenazine, both high potency agents. Many patients require treatment with an anti-EPS agent by mouth when taking depot form antipsychotics.

Answers • 1-C 2-C 3-D

CASE PRESENTATION

A 32-year-old male is being treated with paroxetine 20 mg orally each day for major depressive disorder. He is dependent on nicotine but has no other substance abuse history. After six weeks on the medication, the patient has experienced an improvement in sleep, appetite, and mood. His only remaining complaint is that his interest in having sex with his wife is "lower than ever."

1. The most likely cause for the patient's recent diminished libido is:
   A. Worsening depression
   B. Paroxetine side effects
   C. Spectatoring
   D. An undiagnosed anxiety disorder
   E. None of the above

2. The patient tells you that restoration of sexual functioning is very important to him. The next appropriate step is:
   A. Refer the patient and his wife for couples' therapy
   B. Immediately discontinue paroxetine and start bupropion
   C. Taper paroxetine over 7 to 10 days while adding bupropion
   D. Taper paroxetine over 7 to 10 days while adding venlafaxine
   E. Add sildenafil as needed

3. When initiating selective serotonin re-uptake inhibitors (SSRI) in patients with significant anxiety one should consider:
   A. Starting at relatively low doses of SSRI and slowly titrating upwards
   B. Prescribing clonazepam for a short period (2 to 5 weeks) until anxiety is under control
   C. Prescribing buspirone for a short period (2 to 5 weeks) until anxiety is under control
   D. A and B
   E. A and C

COMMENT

Antidepressants often induce sexual dysfunction • Antidepressant treatment is often beset with sexual side effects. Sexual side effects can be problematic to assess because patients usually do not volunteer information about sexual problems, and clinicians often are not inclined to ask. Sexual dysfunction is often a symptom of depression as well, making it difficult to find a baseline. This particular patient actually seems to be improving in terms of depressive symptoms, but feels decreased libido is a sign of continued depression, when it is much more likely to be a side effect of the SSRI.

Preserving sexual functioning in depressed patients • Three antidepressant medications, bupropion, nefazodone, and mirtazapine, have been shown to preserve sexual functioning. Bupropion does not effect sexual functioning because it is a noradrenergic and dopaminergic drug with no serotonergic properties. Both nefazodone and mirtazapine are considered to be SSRIs with some noradrenergic effects. The reason sexual function is preserved with these two drugs is that in addition to blockade of the reuptake of serotonin, there is a blockade of the 5HT-2 receptor, which is the receptor believed to mediate sexual dysfunction with SSRIs. Venlafaxine would not be a good choice, because it potentiates norepinephrine, dopamine, and serotonin. Remember when discontinuing an SSRI, it is always important to taper the drug due to serotonin withdrawal syndrome, which leaves the patient feeling nauseated, lethargic, and with "flu-like" symptoms. In an intimacy problem most likely caused by an SSRI side effect, adding sildenafil or initiating couples therapy would not be indicated as a first-line intervention. Another factor that supports the use of bupropion in this particular patient is that the drug has been shown to aid in smoking cessation.

SSRIs and anxiety disorders • SSRIs are helpful for the treatment of depression as well as anxiety disorders. However, if the initial dose is too high, patients can experience a significant increase in anxiety. "Start low and go slow" is the best tactic. Low dose, long-acting benzodiazepines can be used on a short-term basis as adjunctive anxiolytic treatment, while antidepressant medications are being titrated slowly upwards. Buspirone, a medication only indicated for generalized anxiety disorder, often takes weeks to start working and therefore would be an inappropriate short-term adjunctive agent.

Answers • 1-B 2-C 3-D

CASE PRESENTATION

A 20-year-old male presents to the emergency room with sudden onset of left hemiplegia and a right frontotemporal headache. The patient had no prior history of any medical problems or family history or risk factors for cardiovascular disease. At the time of examination in the ER, the patient exhibited nystagmus and was somewhat confused though alert and oriented. Patient's blood pressure was 150/110, temperature 99.8 degrees, and pulse was 120. His breath smells of alcohol and the friend who brought him to the ER reports they were drinking and getting high earlier that evening in an abandoned house.

1. The ER physician should:
   A. Reassure the patient that everything will be fine soon and send him home with family support
   B. Order a metabolic panel
   C. Put the patient on a ventilator
   D. Inquire specifically about drug use and order urine toxicology and alcohol breathalyzer test
   E. Observe the patient for 24 hours to see if further problems arise

2. The drug most likely to be responsible for hemiplegia is:
   A. PCP
   B. Cocaine
   C. Alcohol
   D. Marijuana
   E. Nicotine

3. Initial management should include:
   A. A CT scan
   B. Establishing good intravenous access
   C. Stabilizing vital signs if necessary
   D. An electrocardiogram
   E. All of the above

4. The combination of alcohol and cocaine is potentially more dangerous than cocaine alone because:
   A. Alcohol increases cocaine levels in the blood
   B. Cocaine potentiates the pharmacodynamic effects of alcohol
   C. Combination of alcohol and cocaine results in the formation of cocaethylene
   D. It is more expensive to use both alcohol and cocaine
   E. Alcohol causes a more intense "cocaine crash" after cessation of cocaine use

COMMENT

Ask then test • Do not assume that alcohol is the only substance involved. His symptoms further suggest this. Be sure to check a urine drug screen in addition to his alcohol level.

Prime suspect • The patient has probably ingested alcohol together with either intranasal powder cocaine, or more likely, smoked crack cocaine. Cocaine causes an increase in blood pressure, pulse, and temperature. Cocaine can also result in stroke or myocardial infarction. Given the patient's age and lack of family history or risk factors, the hemiplegia was most probably due to cocaine use.

Management • Initial management should include supportive medical care, a CT scan to rule out any intracranial hemorrhage, ECG to rule out myocardial infarction, and establishing IV access.

Evil derivative • The combination of alcohol and cocaine is potentially more dangerous due to formation of cocaethylene, which current research has shown to be more toxic than cocaine alone.

Answers • 1-D 2-B 3-E 4-C

CASE PRESENTATION

A 16-year-old male presents to the emergency room on Saturday night with the chief complaint of "not being able to breath" that started suddenly without warning the same evening at a party. The patient is distraught and also complains of heart racing. The symptoms have occurred a couple of times previously and last about 10 to 20 minutes. There is no prior medical history and the patient's blood pressure is 145/90 with a pulse of 110/minute. Electrocardiogram shows sinus tachycardia and pulse oximetry shows oxygen saturation of 98%.

1. As an emergency room physician, the next intervention should be:
   A. Start IV antihypertensive medication
   B. Intubate the patient
   C. Inquire if the patient ingested any drugs or alcohol at the party
   D. Tell the patient he is malingering
   E. Admit the patient to the hospital

2. The best test to order would be:
   A. Cardiac enzyme levels (CPK)
   B. Chest x-ray to rule out foreign body in the trachea
   C. Urine drug screen and alcohol breathalyzer test
   D. CBC with differential
   E. Amylase level

3. If the urine drug screen comes back positive, which is the most likely drug involved?
   A. Alcohol
   B. Marijuana
   C. Barbiturate
   D. Steroid
   E. Benzodiazepine

COMMENT

Get more information • Given the history, EKG, and vital signs, the next reasonable step would be to ask about substance abuse. The presentation is typical of a patient having a panic attack secondary to illicit drug ingestion at the party. The symptoms of a panic attack include: palpitations, choking sensation, sweating, trembling, chest pain, nausea, dissociative feelings, tingling numbness periorally and in the extremities, chills or hot flushes, and fear of dying or going crazy. The symptoms usually start spontaneously and last about 10 minutes.

Test after asking • Even if the patient denies use of substances at the party, it is wise in this situation to order a urine drug screen and blood alcohol level or alcohol breathalyzer. The patient may not be telling the truth or could have been given a substance unknowingly.

Primary suspect • Marijuana has been implicated in panic attacks, especially among novice users. Most routine urine toxicology exams do not test for steroids.

Answers • 1-C   2-C   3-B

CASE PRESENTATION

A 47-year-old Caucasian woman presents with the chief complaint of chronic back pain at her initial visit to a primary care outpatient office. Patient has been on disability for chronic back pain for the past two years. The patient says her back pain started after an accident at work and that she has been through many procedures and medications for the pain. The patient says she got hooked on pain medicines and wants to stop taking them but has been unsuccessful. She describes a past history of IV heroin use and alcohol abuse. She also has been drinking socially for the past several years and smokes about one pack of cigarettes per day. Except for back pain, her physical exam is unremarkable.

1. Further assessment should include:
   A. Questions about patient's afterlife beliefs
   B. Asking the patient more information about the accident to find out if the pain is real or not
   C. An MRI scan of the head and back
   D. A sleep deprived EEG
   E. Ascertaining which medications the patient is "hooked on" and the duration and amount of medication used, and consider a urine toxicology test

2. The primary care physician should:
   A. Switch her to a new NSAID medication
   B. Tell patient to stop the pain medication after the visit and come back to the clinic next month
   C. Refer the patient to an inpatient detoxification unit familiar with managing pain medication detoxification
   D. Tell the patient there are no other options available currently
   E. Refuse to help the patient until she has a clean UDS

3. The long-term treatment modality that is most effective for the patient's condition is:
   A. Methadone maintenance therapy
   B. Electroconvulsive therapy (ECT)
   C. Naltrexone
   D. Faith-based therapies
   E. Herbal remedies

COMMENT

Ask constructive questions • The patient seems to be dependent on pain medication, most likely an opiate. Intractable chronic back pain and associated medication treatment is commonly involved in iatrogenic opiate dependence.

Proper next step • Given the past history of heroin use, the patient is very likely to relapse to some form of opiate use unless she receives detoxification and rehabilitation in a pain clinic. The patient's care should be coordinated by both the clinician treating her opiate dependence and the clinician involved in pain management.

Medication • Methadone maintenance is the most effective form of long-term treatment for opiate dependence currently available.

Answers • 1-E 2-C 3-A

CASE PRESENTATION

A 40-year-old woman presented to a general medical clinic complaining of times when she experiences palpitations, dizziness, and sweating palms. Upon questioning, it was determined that these symptoms tend to occur when she writes in front of other people such as when she writes her checks at the grocery store and the clerks are watching. She stated the problem has become more pronounced since she recently switched jobs where she is frequently required to write in front of others. At these times her physical symptoms are intolerable and she has started making excuses as to why she cannot write in front of others. She states she fears others will make fun of her if they see her hands shaking when writing. She further revealed that she has passed up certain jobs because of feelings of inadequacy and inferiority and her fear of ridicule from others.

1. Which of the following Axis I diagnoses is most likely?
    A. Specific phobia
    B. Panic disorder
    C. Generalized anxiety disorder
    D. Social phobia
    E. Obsessive-compulsive disorder

2. Which of the following Axis II diagnoses is most likely?
    A. Obsessive-compulsive personality disorder
    B. Dependent personality disorder
    C. Avoidant personality disorder
    D. Schizoid personality disorder
    E. Paranoid personality disorder

3. After reviewing a list of situations that can make some people nervous, the examiner learns that the patient is uncomfortable making presentations and eating in front of others but that she endures these activities despite the discomfort. Given this new information, which specifier might be most appropriate?
    A. Chronic
    B. Severe
    C. Natural environment type
    D. Other type
    E. Generalized

4. Based on surveys of one-year prevalence, which anxiety disorder is the most common?
    A. Specific phobia
    B. Generalized anxiety disorder
    C. Obsessive-compulsive disorder
    D. Social phobia
    E. Posttraumatic stress disorder

COMMENT

Axis I diagnosis • The patient is experiencing social phobia. The most critical symptom in making this diagnosis is her fear of rejection or criticism by others. The physical symptoms listed are common to many anxiety disorders, however, with social phobics, it is the fear of evaluation by others that provokes the anxiety response.

Axis II diagnosis • If the individual fears most social situations, avoids others, has feelings of insecurity and inadequacy, and the pattern is stable across a variety of situations, a diagnosis of avoidant personality is warranted.

Specifier • If the person is afraid of evaluation in multiple situations, the appropriate specifier is "generalized." It is important to thoroughly assess reactions to a variety of social and performance situations.

Most prevalent anxiety disorder • Specific phobia is the most prevalent anxiety disorder

Answers • 1-D 2-C 3-D 4-A

DOG ATTACK

CASE PRESENTATION

Maria is a 23-year-old woman who presented to a clinic with palpitations, fainting, diarrhea, stomach cramps, and a fear that she might be dying. In taking a history, the examiner learns that she was attacked by a dog and hospitalized when she was 12. Since that time she has avoided all places where dogs might attack her. Maria initially feared all large dogs but has recently begun experiencing frequent periods of palpitations, chest pain, dizziness, and a fear that she is dying or having a heart attack. These symptoms reportedly come out of the blue and do not last long. After testing, there appears to be no organic cause for these physical symptoms. She has been able to maintain all daily activities but is doing so with discomfort and fears the physical symptoms might return at any time.

1. Which Axis I disorder is the most likely diagnosis?
   A. Panic disorder with agoraphobia
   B. Specific phobia
   C. Panic disorder without agoraphobia
   D. Generalized anxiety disorder
   E. Delusional disorder

2. If Maria were to develop anxiety about being in places or situations from which escape might be difficult or embarrassing and avoided all public places, which Axis I diagnosis would be most likely?
   A. Panic disorder with agoraphobia
   B. Specific phobia
   C. Panic disorder without agoraphobia
   D. Generalized anxiety disorder
   E. Delusional disorder

3. If these episodes occurred only in the specific, predictable circumstances they would be called:
   A. Phobia responses
   B. Situationally cued
   C. Predispositionally cued
   D. Specifically cued
   E. Environmental responses

4. If when Maria was younger she feared only dogs and attempted to avoid them at all costs, what Axis I disorder would be the most likely diagnosis?
   A. Panic disorders with agoraphobia
   B. Specific phobia
   C. Panic disorder without agoraphobia
   D. Generalized anxiety disorder
   E. Delusional disorder

COMMENT

Axis I disorder • The current presentation of this patient is most consistent with panic disorder without agoraphobia. The physical symptoms of palpitations, fainting, diarrhea, stomach cramps, and a fear that she might be dying are typical of panic attacks. Additionally, the symptoms are coming out of the blue, not only in response to the presence of dogs, and they do not last long. The fear that she might have another panic attack has caused marked distress.

Avoiding public places • If the patient developed anxiety about being in situations from which escape might be difficult and began to avoid such places, this would meet the definition of agoraphobia in addition to the panic attacks.

Specific circumstances • When the attacks are cued by specific, predictable circumstances they are considered to be "situationally cued," because it is the situation that triggers the attacks.

Fear of dogs • Earlier, Maria only feared the presence of dogs, which suggests a specific phobia, animal type. It is only when the fear comes out of the blue and not only in response to dogs that the diagnosis of panic disorder can be considered.

Answers • 1-C 2-A 3-B 4-B

CASE PRESENTATION

Henry is a 28-year-old man who was brought to the clinic by his wife for treatment of his hands. The patient's hands appear to be red, raw, and very irritated. The wife relates that he is washing his hands at least 20 times per day for more than 10 minutes. She stated their marriage has started to suffer as a result of his preoccupation with cleanliness and that although he has always been a perfectionist, he has become "ridiculously perfectionistic" lately. Recently, he has started using bleach to "make sure they get clean" and to be cautious not to be contaminated by germs. He acknowledges that the thoughts about contamination are unwanted and when they occur he washes his hands. He states that when he washes his hands he feels less distressed and can return to his daily activities. The patient reports he isn't really bothered by the thoughts or handwashing behaviors and thinks his wife is overreacting.

1. Which of the following is the most likely Axis I disorder?
   A. Generalized anxiety disorder
   B. Hypochondriasis
   C. Specific phobia
   D. Obsessive-compulsive disorder
   E. Delusional disorder

2. When a patient with this disorder does not seem to be bothered by the symptoms and does not recognize that they are excessive or unreasonable, which specifier is most appropriate?
   A. Acute
   B. Chronic
   C. Poor insight
   D. Delusional
   E. Psychotic features

3. If upon further questioning it was learned that the focus of the patient's fear is that he believes he is interpreting a number of physical symptoms that must be signs of an undiagnosed disease what Axis I diagnosis might better characterize his symptoms?
   A. Generalized anxiety disorder
   B. Hypochondriasis
   C. Specific phobia
   D. Obsessive-compulsive disorder
   E. Delusional disorder

4. What Axis II diagnosis is most likely?
   A. Dependent personality disorder
   B. Borderline personality disorder
   C. Antisocial personality disorder
   D. Obsessive-compulsive personality disorder
   E. Avoidant personality disorder

COMMENT

Axis I disorder • The symptoms presented here are consistent with obsessive-compulsive disorder. The thoughts are unwanted, intrusive, and anxiety producing. As a result, he compulsively washes his hands to reduce the distress.

Specifier • The lack of recognition exhibited by this patient warrants a specifier of poor insight. Patients with obsessive-compulsive disorder often recognize their thoughts are excessive; however, in some cases they lack this insight. The thoughts fall short of being delusional in nature.

Undiagnosed disease • If the focus of the anxiety were about having a serious disease based on the misinterpretation of physical symptoms, then a diagnosis of hypochondriasis might be warranted. If the focus of the anxiety was contracting an illness, then a diagnosis of specific phobia might be warranted.

Axis II disorder • A person who is overly perfectionistic, organized, and rule bound would be diagnosed with obsessive-compulsive personality disorder.

Answers • 1-D 2-C 3-B 4-D

CASE PRESENTATION

Jane Smith, a 28-year-old, married, Caucasian female presents for her first prenatal visit. This is her first pregnancy and she has no chronic health problems. Physical exam is unremarkable except for complaints of nausea and missed menstrual period. She smokes three-quarters to one pack of cigarettes per day and does not participate in any formal exercise. She is 5'4" tall and weighs 118 lbs. She welcomes the new baby, but is uncertain about her ability to quit smoking. "I've tried before, but I always seem to gain weight and I just can't stand that. I have heard that smoking can cause babies to be born smaller. I want my baby to be healthy, but quite frankly, I wouldn't mind if the baby isn't full-size since I don't want to gain weight anyway."

1. According to the federal guidelines for tobacco cessation, as Ms. Smith's physician you should:
   Ask whether or not she is smoking at every visit
   Advise her to quit smoking at every visit
   Assess her readiness to quit smoking
   AND which two?
   A. Announce your readiness to help Ms. Smith in her quit attempt and assist in her quit attempt by providing her with pharmacological and counseling support.
   B. Arouse her interest in quitting by providing motivational literature and assist in her quit attempt by providing her with pharmacological and counseling support.
   C. Avoid nagging her about quitting since this approach can backfire and instead allay her fears about potential harmful effects to the fetus.
   D. Assist in her quit attempt and arrange for follow-up care regarding her smoking status.
   E. Allow Ms. Smith to keep smoking so long as she smokes less than 10 cigarettes per day and has no smoking-related illnesses and ask again at the next visit.

2. Ms. Smith's primary barrier to quitting smoking appears to be weight gain. As her physician, some good advice to give Ms. Smith would be:
   A. "Don't worry about the weight. You'll be gaining approximately 20 lbs. with the pregnancy anyway, what's 5 more pounds?"
   B. "How about starting an exercise program while you quit? Some brisk walking for as little as 15 to 20 minutes per day three days a week would promote blood circulation, which would be beneficial to your baby, and would help keep you from gaining unwanted weight."
   C. "Your biggest concern should be the health of the baby and not how you're going to look in a bathing suit. I suggest you reexamine your priorities."
   D. "A low-calorie, low-fat diet would be a good idea for you while you are trying to quit smoking. At your height and weight, and activity level, you should only need about 1100 to 1200 calories per day."
   E. "A vigorous high-intensity workout program will help you keep from gaining weight and improve your body's composition. An hour per day of aerobic activity each day (e.g., running, biking, stair climbing machine, aerobics class) would certainly do the trick."

3. If Ms. Smith states that she is ready to quit now, which of the following treatments would be most appropriate?
   A. Wellbutrin or nicotine patch plus nicotine inhaler since these are most likely to eliminate weight gain.
   B. Zyban plus clonidine patch, or nicotine patch plus nicotine gum since these methods are best for heavy smokers.
   C. Let Ms. Smith choose her preference from any one of the following: Zyban, nicotine patch, nicotine gum, nicotine nasal spray, or nicotine inhaler.
   D. Nortriptyline or Zyban since both are antidepressants and Ms. Smith may be prone to postpartum depression.
   E. Daily intravenous nicotine injection since it offers a similar bolus of nicotine to the brain that Ms. Smith would obtain from cigarettes without the toxins found in tobacco.

COMMENT

Public Health Service Clinical Practice Guideline • Treating Tobacco Use and Dependence, the Five As: The U.S. Federal Government has developed guidelines for treating tobacco dependence published by the Agency for Health Care Research and Quality in 1996 and updated by the Public Health Service in 2000. The guidelines outline Five As to assist healthcare practitioners in remembering the steps they should practice: ASK every patient if they smoke, if so, ADVISE them to quit, ASSESS their readiness to quit, ASSIST them in their quit attempt, and ARRANGE for follow-up care.

Weight gain after quitting smoking • With respect to the current case, Ms. Smith's concerns about weight gain should be addressed. When prescribing an exercise program, the fact that Ms. Smith is a pregnant beginner should be kept in mind and exercise goals should be accordingly modest. Reducing calories is an appropriate approach for limiting weight gain for a majority of smokers, but given that a pregnant woman is facing increased nutritional needs, this approach is not the best.

Pharmacotherapy for smoking • The first-line pharmacotherapies as listed in the federal guidelines include: Zyban (bupropion hydrochloride) and the nicotine replacement therapies (nicotine patch and nicotine gum, which are available over the counter, and nicotine nasal spray and nicotine inhaler, which are available only by prescription). Clonidine and nortriptyline are second-line pharmacotherapies and should only be considered in cases where the first-line pharmacotherapies have been tried and failed or are contraindicated.

Answers • 1-D 2-B 3-C

TREATING THE OBESE PATIENT

● CASE PRESENTATION

Jennie Jones is a 44-year-old administrative assistant who presents to you at the hypertension clinic. She was referred by her primary care physician who has placed her on antihypertensive medication with good results (current blood pressure: 125/80). She is 5'4" tall and weighs 188 lbs. (BMI = 32; and in the moderately overweight range according to the standard height/weight table); her waist circumference is measured at 38 inches. Her waist to hip ratio is 1.20. She is 26% body fat according to the caliper method of body composition and 28.5% according to the bioelectrical impedance method. Her own medical history is remarkable for appendectomy at age 19. Her LDL cholesterol is 152 mg/dl and her HDL is 40 mg/dl; her fasting plasma glucose is 138 mg/dl. Family history: mother suffers from osteoarthritis, depression, and liver disease. Father has been a type 2 diabetic for many years and underwent bypass surgery at age 49 following myocardial infarction. She has a monozygotic twin with lupus and hypertension. She reports that she gained 12 lbs. after quitting her 25 cigarettes per day habit 18 months ago and does not currently exercise.

1. Which of the following considerations apply to the pharmacological/surgical management of obesity/overweight for Ms. Jones?
    A. She should be offered pharmacotherapy only after lifestyle changes (i.e., dietary habits and physical activity) have been attempted and have not resulted in weight loss after one month.
    B. Because Ms. Jones has three or more obesity-related risk factors and a BMI above 27, she should be offered pharmacotherapy in addition to lifestyle changes if lifestyle changes alone do not produce significant results in six months.
    C. Recommended pharmacological approaches include caffeine/ephedrine combination, orlistat or sibutramine.
    D. Liposuction is a good option for Ms. Jones since she does not exercise, is not morbidly obese, and is not likely to comply with a behavioral weight loss program.
    E. Gastric bypass surgery should be recommended at this point.

2. The best behavioral recommendations for Ms. Jones would be:
    A. Keep a food diary to monitor her caloric intake, incorporate physical activity into existing daily routine (e.g., take stairs instead of elevator, park car further from entrances to buildings and walk more) and use stimulus control.
    B. Reduce fat intake to no more that 10% of daily caloric intake
    C. Reduce daily caloric intake to one-third current level
    D. Stress management
    E. Exercise five to seven times per week for an accumulated total of 90 minutes per day

3. Provided that Ms. Jones is reasonably motivated to lose weight she should:
    A. Be encouraged to lose 30 lbs. in 60 days by cutting calories to one-third of current levels
    B. Be advised to lose 20% of her body weight (38 lbs.) over the next nine months
    C. Be encouraged to develop an exercise program and dietary changes that result in weight loss of one to two lbs. per week to an initial goal of losing 10% of her body weight
    D. Be told that she will be better off if she simply maintains her weight since yo-yo dieting is known to be deleterious over the long haul
    E. Be advised to try behavioral methods only if pharmacological methods fail

● COMMENT

Pharmacological and surgical management of obesity • Ms. Jones has more than three obesity related risk factors: she has elevated fasting serum glucose >126 = diabetes mellitus as in this patient, she has a waist circumference of 38 or more inches (45 or more inches is a risk factor for men), she is hypertensive, she smokes, her HDL is <35, she has impaired fasting glucose, and she has a family history of premature CHD (age 55 for first-degree men, age 65 for first-degree women). An LDL >160 is also a risk factor. Keep in mind that while orlistat and sibutramine are approved by the FDA for the treatment of obesity, caffeine/ephedrine combination is not. Liposuction is not a treatment for obesity, it is a cosmetic surgery. If lifestyle changes do not promote weight loss after six months, drugs should be considered. Pharmacotherapy is limited to those patients who have a BMI >30 or those who have a BMI >27 if concomitant obesity-related risk factors or diseases exist (i.e., hypertension, dyslipidemia, CHD, sleep apnea, type 2 diabetes). If a patient has not lost 4.4 lbs. after four weeks it is not likely that this patient will benefit from the drug. Currently, sibutramine and orlistat are approved by the FDA for long-term use in weight loss. Sibutramine is an appetite suppressant that is proposed to work via norepinephrine and serotonergic mechanisms in the brain. Orlistat inhibits one-third of fat absorption from the intestine. Both of these drugs have side effects. Sibutramine may increase blood pressure and induce tachycardia; orlistat may reduce the absorption of fat-soluble vitamins and nutrients. These drugs are not FDA approved: phentermine, fenfluramine (withdrawn), leptin, dexfenfluramine (withdrawn), ephedrine plus caffeine and fluoxetine (not approved for obesity), and herbal treatments. Mazindol, diethylpropion, phentermine, benzphetamine, and phendimetrazine are approved for short-term treatment of obesity. Surgery is an option for well-informed and motivated patients who have clinically severe obesity (BMI >40 or a BMI >35) and serious comorbid conditions.

Behavioral and psychological management of obesity • Monitoring intake is one of the most effective behavioral strategies for reducing weight. Stress management, stimulus control, problem solving, contingency management, cognitive restructuring, and social support are other nonpharmacological interventions that are recommended. Patients should be encouraged not to be overly restrictive in calorie and fat intake. While exercise is a key component of weight loss programs, sedentary women like Ms. Jones should be eased into exercise and not given overly ambitious goals at the start. Stress management is a good idea for most people, but is not the most effective way to achieve weight loss.

Setting goals for weight loss • Federal guidelines suggest that the best initial goal for weight loss in obese and overweight individuals is to reduce calories by reducing caloric intake by 500 to 1000 calories per day (not less than 800 cal/day); recommended 1000 to 1200 calories per day for women, 1200 to 1600 calories per day for men with an initial goal to lose 10% of current weight at a rate of 1 to 2 lbs. per week.

Answers • 1-B 2-A 3-C

STRESS MANAGEMENT

● CASE PRESENTATION

Harvey Hardhead, a 62-year-old retired mechanic, is visiting you for management of his diabetes. His blood sugar has been poorly controlled of late and Mr. Hardhead explains why, "I'm too busy to pay it much attention. Our 2-year-old granddaughter has just come to live with us since our daughter has been strung out on pills and alcohol and isn't taking proper care of her. We do the best we can.... I've gone back to work full-time as a cashier at McDonald's to help out with the extra expenses and my wife is doing what she can while taking care of her parents who live on our property in their trailer. I've noticed that my blood pressure is up the last few times I took it at the grocery store. I am aggravated that we have had to take money out of savings to pay for rehab for my daughter and daycare for little Sara. I've been taking some of my daughter's nerve pills and they help me to get a good night's sleep which otherwise I couldn't get, but I am afraid of doing that too often 'cause I don't want to get addicted. Plus, I'm not sure how they might affect my asthma." You notice that Mr. Hardhead has difficulty hearing you and upon further examination you conclude that he is suffering from hearing loss associated with old age. You also notice that Mr. Hardhead has lost approximately 15 lbs. since his last visit six months ago.

1. Which of the following conditions also reported by Mr. Hardhead is/are likely to be associated with stress?
   A. Increased blood cholesterol
   B. Jaw and/or tooth pain
   C. Decreased libido
   D. Gastrointestinal distress
   E. All of the above

2. Mr. Hardhead has plenty of company. What percentage of patients visiting their health care provider report conditions that can be attributed to stress?
   A. 15 to 20%
   B. 25 to 30%
   C. 40 to 60%
   D. 75 to 90%
   E. Nearly 100%

3. What does the Holmes-Rahe scale measure?
   A. A variety of reflexes that are heightened in response to stress
   B. It lists common stressors that have been assigned numerical values which, when summed, give an indication of the level of stress someone is under.
   C. It is an electromyographic test (EMG) that measures the level of tension in the muscles at standard sites. The higher the summed reading, the greater the level of stress a person is experiencing.
   D. It is a self-report questionnaire in which the respondent indicates how he or she would respond to a hypothetical stressful situation. It gives an indication of the respondent's favored coping strategies.
   E. It is a self-report questionnaire in which the respondent indicates the social supports available to him or her during times of stress.

4. Which of the following interventions would you recommend for Mr. Hardhead to help him with his stress?
   A. Get involved in a support group at church
   B. Problem-solving approaches
   C. Meditation
   D. Join a competitive senior swim team
   E. A, B, and C

● COMMENT

Stress and comorbid conditions • Stress has been shown to affect almost all body systems, resulting in cardiovascular disease, neuromuscular disorders (including headaches and chronic back pain), respiratory and allergic disorders, immunologic disorders, gastrointestinal disturbances (including peptic ulcer disease, irritable bowel syndrome, nausea, vomiting, and diarrhea), skin diseases, dental problems, and a host of other disorders. Stress causes the adrenal glands to increase production of glucocorticoids (cortisol, cortisone, and catecholamines). These hormones are essential for the metabolism of glucose. Stress can cause sugar to be released into the bloodstream and aggravate diabetes. Other symptoms of stress include reduced production of sex hormones, which can result in decreased sex drive and, in women, irregular or absence of a menstrual cycle. Stress can also cause dry mouth and increased blood cholesterol.

Prevalence of stress • 75 to 90% of patients visiting their health care provider report conditions that can be attributed to stress.

Assessing factors that contribute to stress • The Holmes-Rahe scale attempts to identify life events that typically result in stress and assign a numerical score to each one. When the scores associated with each of the stressors occurring in a person's life are summed, the total is an estimate of how much stress a person is experiencing.

Strategies for stress management • A great way to help Mr. Hardhead learn to alleviate some stress is by helping him generate solutions to the problems that are causing stress, like his financial problems or caring for his daughter. You can also help by recommending or teaching him good relaxation strategies such as meditation, progressive muscle relaxation, visualization, and deep breathing. Increasing his social support network through his church, family, or friends is also highly recommended. Assuming a leadership role of any kind is stressful and is not indicated for someone who is already under significant stress. While physical activity can help alleviate stress, joining a competitive team is likely to put even more pressure on Mr. Hardhead and is not indicated.

Answers • 1-C 2-D 3-B 4-E

CASE PRESENTATION

A psychiatrist sees three new patients in a day. Two of the new patients, Jorge and Carlisle, seem to have panic disorder. The third patient, Allie, seems to have generalized anxiety. However, by doing a review of systems, the psychiatrist recognizes that an underlying medical condition is involved in all three cases.

1. Jorge presents with sudden onset of severe anxiety and irritability. However, he also has associated headaches, diaphoresis, and visual blurring. Recently, he found his blood pressure is elevated (210/140) during these episodes. The most likely explanation for his symptoms is:
   A. Temporal arteritis
   B. Migraine headache
   C. Pheochromocytoma
   D. Alcohol withdrawal
   E. Essential hypertension

2. Carlisle presents with episodes of sudden onset of severe anxiety, severe mood swings, and outbursts of anger. She has also been having abdominal pain and vomiting. She has a peripheral neuropathy and a long history of photosensitivity. The most likely cause of her anxiety is:
   A. Migraine headache
   B. Eczematoid dermatitis
   C. Neuroleptic side effect
   D. Acute intermittent porphyria
   E. Menopause

3. Allie presents with a more constant and less intense form of anxiety. She seems "hyper" and is tremulous. She has heat intolerance, frequent diaphoresis, and warm, moist skin. She has also been losing weight lately. The most likely cause of her symptoms is:
   A. Attention deficit disorder
   B. Hyperthyroidism
   C. Cocaine dependence
   D. Hypoglycemia
   E. Nicotine dependence

COMMENT

Catecholamine-induced hypertension • A marked elevation in blood pressure along with the other symptoms suggests pheochromocytoma. The diagnosis can be confirmed by checking for elevated levels of serum catecholamines and their metabolites in the urine.

Vampires? • It is thought that, in the Middle Ages, people with acute intermittent porphyria may have inspired the story of vampires. These people would stay indoors during the day and come out only at night, due to their photosensitivity. Their mood swings and anger made them feared.

Remember the thyroid • These are all symptoms of hyperthyroidism.

Answers • 1-C 2-D 3-B

CASE PRESENTATION

Fred is a 51-year-old male with alcohol dependence who has been your patient for several years. He typically drinks 6 to 12 beers per day and has fallen on hard times. His use of alcohol has caused significant problems in terms of his ability to work and keep a job, and this in turn has led to financial problems. His limited income puts him below the poverty level.

1. Fred presents to your office complaining of insomnia. He looks depressed and seems more irritable than usual. You note he is having problems with his memory and has "restless legs." His lab work reveals a low hematocrit. The most likely cause of his symptoms is:
   A. Major depression
   B. Hepatic encephalopathy
   C. Wernicke-Korsakoff syndrome
   D. Folate deficiency
   E. Iron deficiency

2. The following year, you see Fred again. He again seems irritable and depressed but more apathetic than before. He has ataxia, atrophic glossitis, and has lost weight. The most likely cause of his symptoms is:
   A. B_{12} deficiency
   B. Folate deficiency
   C. Major depression
   D. Aplastic anemia
   E. Bulimia nervosa

3. One year later, Fred presents again with irritability and depression. He is also complaining of a headache. He seems confused but has no other symptoms. He was hired a few days ago to clean out some gutters and fell off a ladder. The most likely cause of his symptoms is:
   A. Cerebellar ataxia
   B. Hepatic encephalopathy
   C. Wernicke's encephalopathy
   D. Subdural hematoma
   E. Factitious disorder

COMMENT

Alcohol-related anemia • Anemia is a common finding in people with alcohol dependence. It could be a result of bone marrow suppression, but when combined with memory disturbances and particularly restless leg syndrome, folate deficiency is the likely cause. Depression/irritability may also be symptoms. Anemia is not a symptom of depression or hepatic encephalopathy.

Tongue involvement • Glossitis is a key finding that points to pernicious anemia, which is one potential cause of a B_{12} deficiency. A macrocytic anemia in association with neurologic symptoms also indicates a B_{12} deficiency. Depression and irritability may also be seen.

Head goes to ground • Intoxicated people are much more likely to have accidents than those who are sober. This is in part due to poor judgment and delayed reactions. A slow response to using the arm to cushion a fall raises the risk of a head injury. Chronic subdural hematomas are not uncommon in people with alcohol dependence, and should be considered in these patients with headaches, confusion, and even a vague or seemingly insignificant history of trauma.

Answers • 1-D 2-A 3-D

● **CASE PRESENTATION**

Gloria, a 30-year-old female, presents to the office complaining of depression, fatigue, weight loss, and joint pain. Physical exam reveals lymphadenopathy and a malar rash.

1. The most likely diagnosis is:
   A. Major depression with a comorbid viral infection
   B. Rheumatoid arthritis
   C. Systemic lupus erythematosus
   D. Dermatomyositis
   E. Lymphoma

2. Gloria subsequently begins to exhibit psychotic symptoms. These symptoms are most likely due to:
   A. Initiation of treatment of the illness with radiation
   B. The severity of the depression
   C. The use of illicit drugs to relieve the pain
   D. CNS involvement of the illness
   E. New onset of schizophrenia

3. Treatment with steroids is then initiated. Which of the following disorders could most likely occur as a result?
   A. Psychotic disorder
   B. Eating disorder
   C. Attention deficit disorder
   D. Personality disorder
   E. Body dysmorphic disorder

● **COMMENT**

A great imitator • Systemic lupus erythematosus (SLE) is a disease that can present with a variety of symptoms, including all of the symptoms mentioned. Systemic complaints including fever, fatigue, and weight loss are common. Involvement of the CNS may manifest in subjective complaints of depression or cognitive impairment. A malar (butterfly) or discoid rash are classic skin manifestations of SLE. SLE is commonly seen in women (10:1 over men) with onset frequently occurring in the second or third decade of life.

Lupus cerebritis • Approximately 30% of patients with SLE will have involvement of the CNS, which may then lead to psychosis. This may occur with or without the presence of depression.

Steroid-induced psychosis • Large doses of corticosteroids are sometimes used for severe cases of SLE, especially those with CNS or renal manifestations. Unfortunately, these high doses can cause a psychotic reaction, which can be difficult to distinguish from the psychosis induced by the illness itself. A temporal relationship between the onset of treatment with steroids and the onset of psychotic symptoms is helpful in trying to make this distinction, but a reduction in the dose of steroids may also be necessary if possible.

Answers • 1-C 2-D 3-A

CASE PRESENTATION

A 68-year-old man has a 10-year history of suboptimally controlled diabetes mellitus, and now complains of a six-month history of severe burning pain involving both feet. The painful burning dysesthesias are particularly severe over the soles of his feet and most noticeable when the patient attempts to fall asleep at night. Neurologic examination is remarkable for distal impairment of pain and temperature sensation to the mid-shin level bilaterally. Proprioception and vibratory sense are preserved. Deep tendon reflexes are present and symmetrical throughout. Distal lower extremity strength is normal. A trial of amitriptyline as treatment for neuropathic pain was initiated at 25 mg by mouth every night at bedtime. The patient became confused one week after initiating this therapy. Amitriptyline was discontinued and the patient's mental status returned to baseline approximately one month later.

1. The most likely etiology for this patient's bilateral lower extremity pain is:
   A. Painful small fiber peripheral neuropathy
   B. Painful large fiber peripheral neuropathy
   C. Distal peripheral ischemia
   D. Factitious disorder
   E. None of the above

2. Neuropathic pain secondary to diabetic peripheral neuropathy may respond to:
   A. Carbamazepine
   B. Tricyclic antidepressants
   C. Gabapentin
   D. Phenytoin
   E. Any of the above

3. Use of first-generation tricyclic antidepressant agents (amitriptyline) in the elderly patient may be primarily limited by:
   A. Bone marrow depression
   B. Limited bioavailability
   C. Anticholinergic toxicity
   D. Cost
   E. Availability in pharmacies

4. Use of the following drugs should be especially avoided in the elderly patient:
   A. Cox-2 inhibitors
   B. Diphenhydramine
   C. Acetaminophen
   D. Amitriptyline
   E. B and D

COMMENT

Etiology • Painful burning dysesthesias are a frequent complication of patients with long-standing diabetes mellitus. Painful peripheral neuropathy is a common clinical manifestation of damage to small myelinated and unmyelinated peripheral nerve fibers. Multiple metabolic abnormalities complicating diabetes mellitus have been implicated in the pathophysiology of painful diabetic peripheral neuropathy. Elevated levels of potentially neurotoxic metabolic intermediates related to abnormal carbohydrate metabolism may be present. Reduced myoinositol levels may also be involved in the pathogenesis of diabetic neuropathy. There is evidence that strict diabetic control may delay the onset of peripheral neuropathy complications.

Effective medications • Numerous agents are available that may improve symptoms of painful peripheral neuropathy. These include tricyclic antidepressants and various anticonvulsant drugs.

Limiting factor • The geriatric patient is more susceptible than young adults to the anticholinergic toxic potential of tricyclic antidepressants. First-generation tricyclic agents as exemplified by amitriptyline are particularly prone to cause anticholinergic toxicity in the older patient. This may be manifested as confusion, blurred vision, or dry mouth. Urinary retention may be particularly troublesome for the elderly male patient.

Avoid use • It is advisable to avoid use of tricyclic antidepressants, which have the potential for causing anticholinergic toxicity in geriatric patients. Alternative agents such as gabapentin, carbamazepine, and phenytoin may be considered, although other factors may limit their use, including cost and the potential for other side effects. This is particularly true for carbamazepine, which has been associated with bone marrow toxicity.

Answers • 1-A 2-E 3-C 4-E

CASE PRESENTATION

An 84-year-old woman with Alzheimer's disease and bone metastases from breast cancer was recently transferred to a nursing home for terminal care. Her recent clinical course had been characterized by frequent intermittent confusion and agitation. Pain assessment has been difficult since the patient had limited ability to communicate the location or severity of pain to the nursing staff. Present pain management includes 60 mg acetaminophen/60 mg codeine as needed every four to six hours. The patient has unpredictable episodes of grimacing, rapid pacing, and groaning, which seem to improve within one to two hours of receiving medication.

1. Pain management of the elderly patient may be compromised by:
   A. Underreporting of pain by the geriatric patient
   B. Difficulty assessing pain in the cognitively impaired elderly patient
   C. Unfounded physician fears of creating opioid addiction in the geriatric patient
   D. A and B
   E. A, B, and C

2. Signs and symptoms of pain in the cognitively impaired elderly patient may include:
   A. Grimacing
   B. Agitated behavior
   C. Delirium
   D. Pacing aimlessly about the room
   E. All of the above

3. The following pain management modalities may be appropriate for the geriatric patient:
   A. High-dose amitriptyline for neuropathic pain
   B. Nonsteroidal anti-inflammatory agents
   C. Opioids
   D. B and C
   E. All of the above

COMMENT

Limitations to effective pain management • Numerous barriers exist to providing excellence in end-of-life care for the geriatric patient. Major challenges exist in the assessment of pain and providing appropriate pain management for the elderly patient. Geriatric patients often have reduced expectations for pain control, since they may interpret pain as an inevitable consequence of growing old and terminal illness. Doctors have cited fear of creating an addiction as a factor in prescribing opiates, even in dying patients.

Presentation of pain • Frail geriatric patients often have a limited ability to express the intensity and frequency of their pain. Cognitively impaired patients often express pain by grimacing, frowning, fidgeting, or groaning. A pain assessment instrument utilizing a series of faces, from smiling to frowning, may be more useful than a numerical scale to evaluate pain in the cognitively impaired geriatric patient. In the United States, approximately 20% of patients die in a long-term care facility. Although an estimated 90% of pain can be adequately controlled, studies indicate that between 25 and 40% of long-term care residents experience undertreated or untreated pain.

Effective management • State-of-the-art pain management protocols often utilize regularly scheduled doses of analgesic agents, rather than on an as-needed basis. As-needed dosing of patients with chronic pain is usually inadequate as the primary pain management approach, but may be useful as supplementary therapy for breakthrough pain. The science of pain management has advanced dramatically over the past 10 years. The American Pain Society, The World Health Organization, and Department of Health and Human Services are valuable resources in providing pain management strategies.

Answers • 1-E 2-E 3-D

CASE PRESENTATION

An 87-year-old nursing home resident has moderately advanced probable Alzheimer's disease. Change in mental status was noted in this elderly woman over a 24-hour period. The patient became confused, agitated, and combative. Examination revealed normal vital signs, but with urinary incontinence. She was afebrile. Her physical examination including neurologic assessment was within normal limits except for mini-mental status examination score of 11 out of 30 points possible. Laboratory evaluation included normal serum electrolytes, BUN, and creatinine. WBC 8.6 (84 polys, 14 lymphs, 2 monos); hematocrit 35, normal RBC indices. Urinalysis included WBCs, too many to count; 10 to 20 RBCs, and many bacteria. Culture grew >100,000 *E. coli*, sensitive to trimethoprim sulfa. The patient's mental state improved two weeks following initiation of antibiotic therapy.

1. The patient's clinical presentation is consistent with a diagnosis of:
   A. Sensory deprivation
   B. Delirium
   C. Wernicke's encephalopathy
   D. B and C
   E. None of the above

2. The etiology of delirium may be related to:
   A. Reduced central nervous system cholinergic neuronal reserve
   B. Schizophrenia
   C. Impaired central cholinergic transmission
   D. A and C
   E. None of the above

3. Common causes of delirium affecting the geriatric patient include:
   A. Medications
   B. Fecal impaction
   C. Urinary tract infection
   D. Pneumonia
   E. All of the above

4. Management of acute delirium in the geriatric patient includes:
   A. Identification and removal of the offending agent
   B. Treatment of identifiable underlying causes
   C. Commitment to a psychiatric unit
   D. Dialing 911 for transfer to nearest emergency department
   E. A and B

COMMENT

Diagnosis • Change in mental status occurs frequently in the frail, elderly population. This presentation is consistent with delirium, or an acute confusional state that is caused by an underlying medical condition. The presence of new physical symptoms is suggestive that the confusion may be the result of a delirium.

Etiology • Delirium is a syndrome that can result from many different, unrelated causes. Impaired central cholinergic transmission is considered to be a key underlying factor in the pathophysiology of delirium.

Specific causes • Urinary tract infection is a common cause of delirium in the elderly female resident residing in a long-term care facility. Other common causes of delirium in the geriatric population include pneumonia, acute myocardial infarction, fecal impaction, or metabolic abnormalities including hypo- or hypernatremia, hypercalcemia, and others. Medications having potent anticholinergic toxicity profiles are also a common cause of delirium in geriatric patients. In approximately 50% of instances, a specific cause may not be identified.

Management • The delirium generally clears following proper identification and correction of the underlying problem. In some patients, however, a return to baseline may be delayed. Up to one-third of patients may not return to baseline after treatment of delirium even after a six-month period has elapsed. Evaluation of the patient with delirium should include determination of serum electrolytes, BUN, creatinine, and urinalysis following careful general physical and neurologic examination. Chest x-ray may disclose unsuspected pneumonia. Commitment to a psychiatric bed is generally not indicated since the underlying problem is a medical one.

Answers • 1-B 2-D 3-E 4-E

Section 3

Neurology

Susan M. Brown, MD
Timothy D. Carter, MD
Vanessa K. Hinson, MD, PhD
Jerome E. Kurent, MD, MPH

WEAK, PAINFUL LEGS

CASE PRESENTATION

A 38-year-old male presents complaining of pain in his legs and difficulty walking up stairs. He reports the problem started insidiously within the last two to three months and seems to be gradually worsening. He describes aching pain in his thighs which is worsened by exertion. He has noted increasing difficulty going up and down stairs. He has no other medical problems, but was started on atorvastatin for hypercholesterolemia six months ago after a check-up. There is no family history of similar problems or neurologic disease, but a strongly positive family history for severe coronary artery disease. His exam is remarkable for weakness of hip and knee flexion and extension with relatively normal strength of ankle movements. There is some questionable weakness of the shoulders, but the remainder of his examination is unremarkable.

1. Isolated proximal muscle weakness is most commonly associated with which of the following?
   A. Muscle disease
   B. Peripheral neuropathy
   C. Spinal cord compression
   D. Stroke

2. The best single initial test in this case would be:
   A. Serum creatine phosphokinase (CPK) measurement
   B. Nerve conduction studies and electromyography
   C. MRI of the cervical and thoracic spinal cord
   D. CT scan of the brain

3. Which of the following is true?
   A. A negative family history excludes a genetically based neuromuscular disease
   B. Inflammatory muscle problems are rare in this age group
   C. Statins have not been associated with muscle problems
   D. None of the above
   E. A and B only

4. Further evaluation of this patient reveals a CPK level of 15 times the upper limit of normal. Appropriate measures to consider at this point include which of the following?
   A. Nerve conduction studies and electromyography (NCS/EMG)
   B. Muscle biopsy
   C. Evaluating his renal function
   D. Treating symptomatically with NSAIDs and rechecking CPK in three months
   E. A, B, and C

COMMENT

Differential diagnosis of proximal weakness • Proximal muscle weakness, especially when symmetric, is usually associated with muscle disease. Defects of neuromuscular transmission, such as myasthenia gravis, may also cause weakness that is greater proximally than distally. Peripheral neuropathies generally tend to cause distal muscular weakness and atrophy. Spinal cord compression causes weakness of muscle groups supplied by the portion of the cord at and caudad to the level of compression. Weakness secondary to stroke is most commonly unilateral.

Diagnostic approach to muscle disease • Damaged muscle cells release creatine phosphokinase (CPK) and aldolase, raising serum levels of these enzymes. These lab tests are easily obtainable and relatively inexpensive, making them the best first choice in this case, since the clinical exam suggests a myopathic process. Nerve conduction studies and electromyography (NCS/EMG) may also be useful in helping to narrow the differential diagnosis. The examination is not suggestive of a problem affecting the central nervous system, thus imaging of the brain or spinal cord with either CT or MRI is not likely to be helpful.

Causes of myopathy • Genetically based muscle disease (muscular dystrophies), may have onset at any age and family history may not always be positive. Inflammatory muscle diseases such as polymyositis and dermatomyositis may occur at all ages, although dermatomyositis is more common in children and young adults. Drugs can cause myopathies and this is a well-documented adverse effect of the statins. While this complication can occur with any of the statins, cerivastatin has been recently removed from the market because of excess cases of rhabdomyolysis, renal failure, and death. Myositis may be caused by viral, bacterial, or parasitic sources. Finally, metabolic problems such as thyrotoxicosis, and other inflammatory conditions such as sarcoidosis may be associated with myopathy.

Initial management of myopathy • Further diagnostic testing in this patient would appropriately include NCS/EMG testing and muscle biopsy to confirm the diagnosis. Since muscle injury may potentially lead to myoglobinuria and renal failure, evaluation of renal function is necessary. Statins have been associated with rhabdomyolysis and should be stopped immediately. Merely treating the pain and rechecking only his CPK in a few months is inappropriate since inflammatory and toxic myopathies can lead to progressive disability, renal failure, or even death.

Answers • 1-A 2-A 3-D 4-E

CASE PRESENTATION

A 12-year-old girl is brought to the emergency department because of difficulty speaking. She was well until that morning when her parents noted that she was having trouble speaking and getting dressed for school. She had previously been healthy and there is no history of prenatal or perinatal problems. On exam, she is alert and able to follow most commands, but has difficulty with word finding and decreased fluency of speech. There is flattening of the nasolabial fold on the right and weakness of the right arm.

1. Stroke in children is most commonly related to:
   A. Hypertension
   B. Premature atherosclerosis
   C. Structural heart defects
   D. Vasculitis
   E. None of the above

2. Which one of the following conditions is most commonly associated with stroke in young patients?
   A. Sickle cell anemia
   B. Sickle cell trait
   C. Varicella
   D. Mononucleosis

3. Which of the following statements regarding stroke in children is true?
   A. The prognosis for recovery is worse than adults
   B. Children with homocystinuria are at increased risk for stroke
   C. Children with mitochondrial disease are not at increased risk for stroke
   D. Moyamoya disease is not associated with stroke
   E. All of the above
   F. None of the above

4. In children with sickle cell anemia:
   A. Stroke is uncommon
   B. Screening with MRI may predict risk of stroke
   C. Chronic transfusion therapy is indicated in all children with sickle cell disease to decrease risk of stroke
   D. Aspirin has been proven to decrease stroke risk
   E. None of the above

COMMENT

Differences between stroke in children and adults • While hypertension and atherosclerosis are common risk factors for stroke in adults, they are rarely associated with stroke in children. Vasculitis may cause stroke at any age, but is relatively uncommon. Structural (usually congenital) heart defects may lead to cardioembolic stroke and are a leading cause of stroke in children.

Causes of stroke in children • In addition to congenital heart defects, other inherited conditions including sickle cell anemia, homocystinuria, mitochondrial disorders, and coagulopathies are associated with stroke in young patients. Elevated levels of homocysteine are also associated with vascular risk in adults. Moyamoya disease is an occlusive vasculopathy affecting larger vessels around the Circle of Willis leading to recurrent strokes. While stroke may complicate infectious problems such as varicella, this is uncommon.

Neural plasticity • Plasticity refers to the brain's ability to change or recover in response to a stimulus or injury. Neural plasticity is maximal during infancy and early childhood and decreases with aging. Thus, younger patients generally achieve better recoveries from cerebral insults than adults. For example, hemispherectomy is an accepted treatment for infants roughly under 1 year of age with certain types of refractory seizure disorders. Children treated in such a manner do remarkably well over time, frequently exhibiting only mild hemiparesis as teenagers.

Prevention of stroke in sickle cell anemia • Unfortunately, stroke is not uncommon in children with sickle cell disease. Transcranial doppler ultrasound may be used to select children with sickle cell disease at increased risk for stroke based on elevated flow velocities in the middle cerebral arteries. It has been shown that the risk of first stroke in such children can be decreased by recurrent blood transfusion to decrease the level of sickle hemoglobin. While MRI may be useful diagnostically in individual cases, it has no demonstrated predictive value for stroke in sickle cell patients.

Answers • 1-C   2-A   3-B   4-E

CASE PRESENTATION

A 76-year-old male is brought into the office by his wife who complains he has episodes of confusion. The patient reports the episodes begin with a "funny feeling" in his stomach during which time he reports he experiences a smell of burned rubber. He is unsure what follows over the next few minutes, but notes he feels tired following these events. His wife notes that during the episode, the patient perseverates, smacks his lips in a chewing-like motion, and has difficulty following commands. The confusion lasts two to three minutes, followed by fatigue that lasts a few hours.

1. The following best describes this type of seizure:
   A. Absence
   B. Generalized tonic-clonic
   C. Complex partial
   D. Simple partial
   E. Epilepsia partialis continua

2. The anatomical location of this type of seizure is:
   A. Frontal lobe
   B. Temporal lobe
   C. Occipital lobe
   D. Brainstem
   E. Spinal cord

3. What are possible etiologies for these seizures?
   A. Idiopathic
   B. Trauma
   C. Mesial temporal lobe sclerosis
   D. Congenital brain malformation
   E. All of the above

4. The most likely cause of new onset partial seizures in an elderly person is:
   A. Stroke or tumor
   B. Metabolic derangement
   C. Fever
   D. Delirium
   E. An idiopathic seizure syndrome

COMMENT

Seizure types • Partial seizure refers to a seizure that is activated by neurons limited to part of one cerebral hemisphere whereas generalized seizures are initiated by generalized neuronal activation. Partial seizures may become secondarily generalized if the epileptic activity spreads from the initial area of onset to involve both cerebral hemispheres. If consciousness or responsiveness is impaired during a partial seizure, it is classified as a complex partial seizure. Simple partial seizures are accompanied by normal states of awareness. Absence seizures consist of sudden interruption in activity, a blank stare, and unresponsiveness, which last less than a minute. An absence seizure stops as quickly as it started, then the person resumes normal behavior. The patient is described as having a brief seizure, so this is not epilepsia partialis continua, which refers to refractory partial seizures (usually simple partial) that may last for hours, days, or months.

Localization of seizure types • The aura (premonition) of an unpleasant smell and epigastric discomfort combined with lip smacking, confusion, and repetitive speech are typical of temporal lobe seizures. Occipital seizures are accompanied by simple visual hallucinations. Frontal lobe seizures are accompanied by gestural automatisms at onset and tonic (extension) or postural motor manifestations. The brainstem and spinal cord do not generate seizures as a rule.

Causes of seizures • Any of the etiologies listed for question 3 apply, including focal temporal lobe changes, which are often associated with epilepsy (mesial temporal lobe sclerosis).

New onset seizures in the elderly • In an elderly person, stroke and/or tumor are the most likely etiologies of new onset seizures. These patients should be aggressively studied (primarily with neuroimaging, preferably MRI) until the source is identified or serious underlying pathology is excluded.

Answers • 1-C 2-B 3-E 4-A

CASE PRESENTATION

A 24-year-old female presents to the emergency room with severe right-sided head pain for 12 hours. Before the headache, she reported a short period of having blind spots in her visual fields that subsequently resolved. The onset of the headache was relatively rapid, with little response to acetaminophen and ice. She reports nausea, sensitivity to light, and more frequent occurrence of these headaches with timing of her menses. She has intermittently had similar headaches over the last five years. She requests narcotics for immediate relief of her symptoms. Her physical exam is unremarkable with the exception of a right pupil that is 2 mm larger than the left.

1. What type of headache does this patient have?
   A. Temporal arteritis
   B. Tension headache
   C. Migraine with aura
   D. Cluster headache
   E. Analgesic rebound headache

2. What medications would be more useful than repeated narcotic use in this case?
   A. Valproic acid (Depakote) daily prophylaxis if similar headaches occur more than two times per week
   B. Sumatriptan (Imitrex) with the onset of head pain and repeated in two hours if needed for immediate headache relief
   C. Oxygen inhalation therapy during the course of the headache
   D. Pilocarpine eye drops
   E. A and B

3. What history would indicate additional testing needs to be done?
   A. HIV exposure
   B. Increasing frequency and severity of headache symptoms accompanied by nausea and vomiting and papilledema on exam
   C. Head pain worsening with coughing and exertion
   D. First onset of headache in a patient older than 35 years old
   E. All of the above

4. Which statement about headaches is false?
   A. Migraine headaches have a higher prevalence in women after puberty, but occur equally in boys and girls before puberty
   B. The risk for future stroke is higher in women who are over 35 years old, experience migraine with aura, smoke cigarettes, and use oral contraceptives
   C. The pain of migraine headache is mediated largely by the trigeminal nerve
   D. Migraine headaches do not tend to run in families

COMMENT

Differential diagnosis of headache • Typical symptoms of migraine include a unilateral, moderate to severe headache lasting two to 72 hours, accompanied by nausea, vomiting, photophobia, and/or phonophobia. They are often familial and associated with hormonal changes. Symptoms of migraine may be bilateral and are aggravated by physical activity. Migraine aura consists of premonitory focal, neurologic symptoms that may include visual, sensory, motor, or brainstem (vertigo) dysfunction within one hour of headache onset. While compression of the oculomotor nerve by a mass lesion such as an aneurysm may cause anisocoria, it is not uncommon for migraine patients to have a mydriatic pupil on the side of the head pain.

Tension-type headache classically is described as constant pressure in a band-like distribution around the head. Cluster headaches are severe, periorbital headaches of short duration, associated with ipsilateral conjunctival injection and nasal congestion which occur in periodic clusters. Temporal arteritis is an inflammatory condition associated with headache that affects primarily elderly patients. Analgesic rebound headache is a form of daily headache experienced by patients who take large quantities of analgesics.

Treatment of migraine headache • Before initiating medications for migraine, lifestyle factors (e.g., regular sleep, caffeine, triggers, stress management) should be considered. Rescue, or immediate, therapy for migraine pain typically includes acetaminophen, NSAIDS, aspirin, or over-the-counter migraine medications. Options for more resistant pain include ergots and triptans, which are specific therapies designed to target serotonin receptors. These rescue medications work best when administered with the onset of aura or head pain. Prophylactic medications such as beta blockers, tricyclic antidepressants, or anticonvulsants are recommended when the patient has frequent migraines or contraindications to rescue medications. Oxygen therapy is indicated for cluster headaches. Eye drops are not necessary as pupillary dilatation will resolve with migraine improvement.

Factors suggestive of serious or life-threatening headaches • Since new-onset headaches in middle-aged or elderly patients are unusual, a secondary cause must be a considered. While HIV patients can still have migraines, they are susceptible to opportunistic infections such as toxoplasmosis, cryptococcus, progressive multifocal leukoencephalopathy, and tumors such as lymphoma. Any neurologic deficit or history of progression should prompt neuroimaging and/or lumbar puncture. Options 3b and 3c describe symptoms of increased intracranial pressure that warrant a CT scan to exclude a mass before attempting a lumbar puncture.

Migraine • Migraine is very commonly familial. The other listed responses are all true.

Answers • 1-C 2-E 3-E 4-D

CASE PRESENTATION

A 63-year-old man presents with a three-year history of slowly progressive incoordination and difficulty writing. Upon examination, there is a masked facies, a 4 Hertz rest tremor in the right hand, as well as mild rigidity of all four extremities, worse on the right. Upon walking the right hand tremor increases, and there is reduced arm swing. The remainder of the neurologic examination is normal.

1. Parkinsonism includes which of the following clinical features?
   A. Tremor
   B. Dyskinesia
   C. Akinesia/bradykinesia
   D. Rigidity
   E. Postural instability
   F. Tremor, akinesia/bradykinesia, rigidity, and postural instability
   G. Tremor, dyskinesia, and rigidity

2. There are multiple etiologies for parkinsonism. In this case, the age of onset, unilateral tremor, and relatively slow disease progression suggest that this particular patient suffers from:
   A. Vascular parkinsonism
   B. Diffuse Lewy body disease
   C. Parkinson's disease
   D. Progressive supranuclear palsy
   E. Multiple system atrophy

3. Which of the following treatments may be helpful in Parkinson's disease?
   A. Haloperidol
   B. Alpha methyldopa
   C. Clozapine
   D. Fluphenazine
   E. Prochlorperazine

4. Which of the following drugs are likely to cause worsening symptoms in this patient and should therefore be avoided?
   A. Carbidopa/levodopa
   B. Metoclopramide
   C. Entacapone
   D. Bromocriptine
   E. Selegiline

COMMENT

Clinical features of parkinsonism • Four cardinal features of parkinsonism are tremor, akinesia (or bradykinesia), rigidity, and postural instability. A parkinsonian tremor occurs primarily at rest, although it may be seen with action. Dyskinesias in parkinsonism are more likely related to treatment, rather than representing a primary part of the disorder.

Differential diagnosis of parkinsonism • Parkinsonism can be caused by a variety of disorders. Parkinson's disease (PD) is the most common form of parkinsonism. PD typically presents in the fifth or sixth decade with initially unilateral symptoms of tremor, bradykinesia, and rigidity. Pathologic features of PD include loss of pigmented neurons in the substantia nigra and the presence of Lewy bodies. Vascular parkinsonism is suggested by such features as a known history of cerebrovascular disease, sudden onset of symptoms, or neurologic signs of stroke on examination. Patients with diffuse Lewy body disease often experience prominent visual hallucinations and dementia. Limited voluntary vertical gaze, but present vertical eye movements on oculocephalic testing (supranuclear gaze palsy) is the hallmark of progressive supranuclear palsy. Patients with multiple system atrophy display prominent dysautonomia.

Treatment of Parkinson's disease • Since many of the features of PD are related to lack of dopamine in the extrapyramidal motor system, replacement therapy with levodopa (a chemical precursor of dopamine that is able to cross the blood-brain barrier where it is converted to dopamine) is the most effective therapy. To avoid side effects, levodopa is administered in combination with carbidopa, which prevents the peripheral decarboxylation of levodopa to dopamine. Bromocriptine, pergolide, ropinirole, and other dopamine agonists are frequently effective therapy for PD. Selegiline, an inhibitor of type B monoamine oxidase, inhibits the catabolism of dopamine, thereby increasing its availability in the brain. Catechol–O–methyltransferase inhibitors such as entacapone also increase the availability of dopamine by inhibiting its catabolism. Anticholinergic agents such as benztropine and trihexyphenidyl may also provide symptomatic benefit in PD. The atypical neuroleptic clozapine has very little influence on the striatonigral portion of the dopaminergic system, and is commonly used to treat psychosis in PD. Alpha methyldopa is used to treat hypertension. The other listed options are dopamine antagonists which may cause worsening of symptoms

Drugs to avoid in Parkinson's disease • Dopamine depleting or blocking drugs, such as metoclopramide, should be avoided in any patient with parkinsonism.

Answers • 1-F 2-C 3-C 4-B

CASE PRESENTATION

A 32-year-old woman arranged an office visit for evaluation of a three-day history of numbness and tingling in both distal lower extremities. She is in excellent health and takes no medication. The patient recovered from a viral upper respiratory infection approximately three weeks ago. There is no history of diabetes mellitus, alcohol use or known toxic exposure. The distal lower extremity numbness and tingling have become more prominent over the past 24 hours and she has also experienced mild lower extremity weakness. She has mild shortness of breath. Neurologic examination demonstrates mild foot dorsiflexor weakness bilaterally, with absent deep tendon reflexes in the upper and lower extremities. Plantar stimulation reveals downgoing toes bilaterally. One day later, she is slightly weaker overall, and mild bilateral facial weakness is present. Objective sensory examination is intact to pin, light touch, temperature, vibration and position.

1. Which of the following are included in the differential diagnosis?
    A. Acute paralytic poliomyelitis
    B. Botulism
    C. Guillain-Barré syndrome (acute inflammatory polyradiculoneuropathy)
    D. Tick bite paralysis
    E. All of the above

2. Complications of Guillain-Barré syndrome may include:
    A. Respiratory failure
    B. Labile blood pressure
    C. Cardiac dysrhythmia
    D. All of the above
    E. None of the above

3. Therapeutic interventions of proven value include:
    A. Corticosteroids
    B. Intravenous IgG
    C. Plasmapheresis
    D. B and C
    E. All of the above

4. The underlying pathophysiology of Guillain-Barré syndrome most often involves the following:
    A. Acute axonal peripheral neuropathy
    B. Inflammatory myopathy
    C. Neuromuscular junction defect
    D. Demyelinating peripheral neuropathy
    E. None of the above

COMMENT

Features of Guillain-Barré syndrome • The Guillain-Barré syndrome (GBS) is an inflammatory demyelinating peripheral neuropathy and frequently has a temporal relationship to antecedent mild viral upper respiratory or gastrointestinal illness. Symptoms of GBS usually occur within three weeks of the viral syndrome. Case fatality rate is approximately 5% and usually is due to respiratory failure, cardiac dysrhythmias, or complications of chronic immobilization and mechanical ventilation. Nerve conduction studies may be normal within the first several weeks of the illness and are of relatively limited value. However, the F wave may be prolonged during the early clinical course. Spinal fluid examination typically reveals an elevated protein level with normal cell counts and other parameters.

Complications of GBS • Dysautonomia may occur frequently and may manifest as labile blood pressure and cardiac dysrhythmias. Heart block may occur on rare occasion. It is particularly important to monitor pulmonary function in patients with suspected GBS. Serial forced vital capacity determination (FVCs) is a useful way of monitoring mechanical pulmonary reserve. Worsening FVCs should prompt prophylactic intubation for ventilatory support in a controlled, rather than emergent, setting.

Treatment of GBS • Plasmapheresis may reduce the period of neuromuscular weakness, and reduce time of recovery if initiated during the first two weeks of clinical presentation. Plasma exchange is usually reserved for patients with moderately severe and rapidly advancing weakness. Corticosteroids are of no value in reducing the severity of symptoms or increasing the rate of neurologic recovery. Intravenous IgG has also been shown to be of value and may be considered if plasmapheresis is not associated with clinical improvement or is unavailable.

Pathophysiology of GBS • A demyelinating peripheral neuropathy is most commonly seen in GBS. Rarely, a primarily axonal neuropathy may be demonstrated electrophysiologically. Demyelination in GBS is thought to be secondary to a monophasic autoimmune process, perhaps triggered by recent antecedent infection. Hepatitis B, HIV, and *Campylobacter* have been implicated in some patients with GBS. However, most patients with GBS do not have a specific infectious agent demonstrated as the cause of their weakness.

Answers • 1-E 2-D 3-D 4-D

CASE PRESENTATION

A newborn, premature (36 weeks gestational age) infant is observed by nursing staff to have apneic spells, temperature instability, and poor feeding. The nurses report that during these spells, the baby has eye fluttering, sucking movements, and tonic posturing. The baby has experienced numerous spells lasting five to 10 minutes each over the last three hours. The child's birth was reportedly uneventful with APGARs of 5 and 8. On exam, all motor functions are symmetrical with reflexes intact. There is a family history of febrile seizures.

1. To determine the cause of neonatal seizures, the following tests should be ordered:
   A. Blood cultures, CBC, urine studies, and lumbar puncture to identify sepsis
   B. Neuroimaging of the brain to look for bleeding
   C. Metabolic studies
   D. Maternal drug screen
   E. All of the above

2. Febrile seizures:
   A. Most commonly start in children 1 month of age or less
   B. Are best treated with anticonvulsant medications after the first seizure
   C. Are more likely to be associated with epilepsy when they are prolonged, recur within 24 hours, or occur in a child with abnormal neurologic status
   D. Do not usually run in families
   E. Are considered simple febrile seizures when they last less than one hour

3. With a diagnosis of neonatal seizures, the best medication would be:
   A. Acetaminophen
   B. Narcan
   C. Phenobarbital
   D. Carbamazepine

4. Inborn errors of metabolism that can cause neonatal seizures are:
   A. Maple syrup urine disease
   B. Carbamyl phosphate synthetase deficiency
   C. Pyridoxine deficiency
   D. Hyperglycinemia
   E. All of the above

COMMENT

Evaluation of neonatal seizures • This baby has some features of normal premature infants: temperature instability, difficulty feeding effectively, and sucking movements. On the other hand, the constellation of symptoms including apneic spells, face or eye movements, and abnormal posturing would indicate pathologic "subtle" neonatal seizures. Common causes of neonatal seizures are hypoxic-ischemic injury, sepsis, premature neonatal brain hemorrhage, hypoglycemia, hypocalcemia, and drug withdrawal. Brain malformations and inborn errors of metabolism should be included in the differential. Testing should include evaluation for all of these diagnostic possibilities. Idiopathic or febrile seizures in neonates are rare. A syndrome that can develop during the first week, associated with apnea, is benign familial neonatal seizures. It is usually a diagnosis of exclusion.

Febrile seizures • Febrile seizures, often familial, usually start between the ages of 3 months and 5 years. Antiepileptic medications administered in the setting of febrile seizures have not proven effective in preventing epilepsy. Two-thirds of children will have a single febrile seizure without further seizures, and therefore, the side effects of medication do not warrant their continued use. Once febrile seizures are accompanied by complex features, such as those listed in answer C, there is a higher likelihood of the child developing afebrile epilepsy.

Treatment of neonatal seizures • Diagnostic and therapeutic procedures should proceed concurrently. Initially, adequate oxygenation and hemodynamic stability should be achieved. Hypoglycemia or other readily identifiable metabolic abnormalities should be promptly corrected. Anticonvulsant therapy should be initiated since continued seizures promote brain irritability and neuronal insult. Phenobarbital is the most commonly used anticonvulsant in this setting. Carbamazepine has no available parenteral formulation and is not appropriate in this setting. Acetaminophen is helpful for reducing fever, which may reduce the seizure threshold. Narcan may be diagnostic for maternal drug transmission, but may further promote an unwanted sudden withdrawal process.

Inborn errors of metabolism • There are many inborn errors of metabolism that can present with seizures. Evaluating serum, urine, and/or CSF for abnormalities such as low glucose, elevated ammonia, elevated lactate, or metabolic acidosis may help to identify a metabolic pathway that has been compromised. All of the listed disorders in this question may cause seizures. While rare, it is important to note that pyridoxine deficiency can result in refractory neonatal seizures and pyridoxine should be given to any infant with seizures that are not controlled with anticonvulsants.

Answers • 1-E 2-C 3-C 4-E

CASE PRESENTATION

A 22-year-old male presents to the emergency room with "the worst headache of my life" beginning four hours ago. The pain is severe over the right parietal area, continuous, and accompanied by right pupil dilatation, right lid weakness, and difficulty moving the right eye nasally. He has no history of headaches, trauma, or significant illness. Physical exam reveals no further neurologic deficits, but the patient complains of mild neck stiffness.

1. What would you expect in subarachnoid hemorrhage?
   A. Identifiable hemorrhage on CT in 90% of cases.
   B. Blood in cerebrospinal fluid (CSF) appearing in the first lumbar puncture tube, but significantly less in tube 4.
   C. Lack of xanthochromia in the CSF at least 24 hours after onset of symptoms.
   D. Improvement of initial symptoms, only to return three to five days later.
   E. A and D
2. Risk factors or disease associations with subarachnoid hemorrhage are:
   A. Trauma and saccular aneurysms
   B. Hypotension
   C. Renal carcinoma
   D. Atrial fibrillation
   E. Hypothyroidism
3. Treatment of subarachnoid hemorrhage includes:
   A. Neurosurgical evaluation for clipping, aneurysm coil placement, or embolization
   B. Nimodipine to prevent subsequent vasospasm
   C. Control of hypertension
   D. Mannitol, hyperventilation, steroids, and shunts to reduce intracranial pressure when indicated
   E. All of the above
4. What complications can arise from SAH?
   A. Rebleeding
   B. Prolongation of QT interval and arrhythmias on EKG
   C. Seizures and focal neurologic deficits
   D. Change in mental status
   E. All of the above

COMMENT

Clinical features and diagnostic evaluation of subarachnoid hemorrhage (SAH) • "The worst headache of my life" of acute onset is a neurosurgical emergency until proven otherwise by a normal CT, lumbar puncture, and physical exam. Cerebrospinal fluid findings frequently include elevated opening pressure and grossly bloody fluid with 100,000 to 1 million plus red blood cells. The amount of blood in the CSF does not significantly decrease as CSF tubes are collected as may be seen with a traumatic LP. Xanthochromia, or yellow pigmentation of the supernatant of centrifuged CSF, is indicative of RBC breakdown from hemorrhage. A subsequent chemical meningitis causes localized nucchal rigidity and irritation. A "sentinel bleed," heralded by an unusual or severe headache, may occur with temporary improvement, only to be followed by subsequent rebleeding and clinical deterioration. Third nerve palsy, presenting with ipsilateral pupil dilatation, ptosis, and restricted extraocular eye movements, may be a presenting feature of posterior communicating artery aneurysms. Once SAH has been diagnosed, the vascular cause of bleeding can best be determined with cerebral angiography, which is used to guide surgical therapy.

Causes of subarachnoid hemorrhage • Subarachnoid hemorrhage, most commonly caused by trauma, ruptured berry aneurysm or arteriovenous malformation rupture, is associated with hypertension, polycystic kidney disease, and cocaine/amphetamine use. Atrial fibrillation is more commonly associated with embolic stroke.

Complications of subarachnoid hemorrhage • Neurologic complications include cerebral vasospasm leading to ischemic brain injury, seizures, hydrocephalus, and mental status changes. Systemic complications include EKG changes, arrhythmias, neurogenic pulmonary edema, hyponatremia, and chemical meningitis due to irritation of the meninges by blood in the subarachnoid space.

Treatment of subarachnoid hemorrhage • Treatment of subarachnoid hemorrhage is neurosurgical in most cases, utilizing microneurosurgical techniques. The less-invasive techniques of arterial embolization, coil placement into the aneurysm via catheter, and/or stereotactic radiosurgery of arteriovenous malformations are being used more frequently in situations not amenable to traditional open surgical techniques. In order to minimize complications, interventions for treating seizures, controlling blood pressure and vasospasm, and reducing increased intracranial pressure should be implemented.

Answers • 1-E 2-A 3-E 4-E

CASE PRESENTATION

A 65-year-old gentleman comes to your office because of complaints of double vision. He has noted intermittent diplopia for about one to two months. He has also noted some occasional difficulties with swallowing and reports he feels tired all of the time. Evenings are especially bad for him and his wife has noted he seems to have difficulty keeping his eyes open at night after supper. He reports he feels best in the mornings. His examination is remarkable for mild bilateral ptosis, subjective complaints of horizontal diplopia on right lateral gaze, and a somewhat nasal voice. The remainder of his physical and neurologic examination is unremarkable.

1. This condition is caused by:
   A. Antibodies to postsynaptic acetylcholine receptors at the neuromuscular junction
   B. Antibodies to presynaptic calcium channels at the neuromuscular junction
   C. Paroxsymal hypokalemia
   D. Autoimmune thyroiditis
   E. An inherited metabolic defect

2. Which of the following is most likely to provide helpful diagnostic information?
   A. MRI of the brain
   B. Referral for ophthalmologic evaluation
   C. Serum electrolytes
   D. Tensilon test
   E. Lumbar puncture

3. This condition may be best treated with:
   A. Potassium supplementation
   B. Immunosuppression
   C. Thyroid ablation with I^{131}
   D. Anticoagulation
   E. Antibiotics

4. After the diagnosis is made, further testing should include:
   A. CT scan of the chest
   B. Electrocardiogram
   C. Echocardiography
   D. Screening for carrier status of asymptomatic relatives
   E. Fasting blood glucose

COMMENT

Diagnosis of myasthenia gravis (MG) • The symptom complex of flucuating diplopia, ptosis, and fatiguability suggests myasthenia gravis (MG). MG is caused by autoimmune destruction of postsynaptic acetylcholine receptors at the neuromuscular junction. Lambert-Eaton myasthenic syndrome (LEMS) is another disease of the neuromuscular junction caused by autoimmune destruction of presynaptic calcium channels. LEMS occurs most commonly as a paraneoplastic syndrome associated with lung cancer.

Diagnostic testing in MG • Administration of a short-acting acetylcholinesterase inhibitor such as edrophonium (Tensilon) can temporarily reverse physical signs of MG such as ptosis. Tensilon may cause bradycardia and should only be administered in a setting where bradycardia can be treated emergently. Cooling the neuromuscular junction also improves neuromuscular transmission so that placing an ice pack over the eye can improve ptosis temporarily as well in these patients. While helpful, neither of these procedures is diagnostic of MG. More definitive diagnostic tests include measurement of antibodies against acetylcholine receptors in the serum, and electrodiagnostic techniques such as repetitive nerve stimulation or single fiber electromyography.

Treatment of MG: • Mild MG may be treated with longer acting acetylcholinesterase inhibitors such as pyridostigmine. Patients who have much symptomatology beyond mild ocular problems usually require treatment with immunosuppressive agents such as prednisone, azathioprine, cyclosporine, or other strategies such as periodic infusion of intravenous immunoglobulin or plasmapheresis. Myasthenic crisis is the relatively acute occurrence of critical weakness of respiratory or bulbar musculature and can be life threatening. It is usually treated with the combination of plasmapheresis and steroids.

Thymectomy for MG • Since MG has been associated with thymoma, patients with MG should have a CT scan of the chest as part of their evaluation. The removal of any residual thymic tissue in MG patients without thymoma may be associated with clinical improvement.

Answers • 1-A 2-D 3-B 4-A

CASE PRESENTATION

A 17-year-old female is brought by EMS to the emergency room for loss of consciousness and convulsions. By report, she has a known seizure disorder and has been seizing for at least 20 minutes. She is febrile, tachycardic, but has a normal blood pressure. Initially, she was noted to have left facial twitching, but now she has bilateral continuous clonic activity. She is not responsive to deep pain. Her cranial nerve exam reveals bilateral pupil dilatation, intact corneal and gag reflexes, and symmetrical facial features. She moves all extremities equally. Bilateral Babinski responses are produced with plantar stimulation. Serum glucose and antiepileptic drug levels have been ordered.

1. After initially achieving cardiopulmonary stability, in what order would you give the following medications to control seizure activity?
   A. Thiamine, narcan, phenobarbital, dextrose, lorazepam
   B. Dextrose, thiamine, narcan, phenytoin, lorazepam
   C. Lorazepam, thiamine, dextrose, narcan, phenytoin
   D. Phenytoin, phenobarbital, dextrose, thiamine, narcan

2. What is the most likely cause of status epilepticus in this patient?
   A. Antiepileptic medication noncompliance
   B. Infections, including meningitis
   C. Trauma (e.g., subdural hematoma)
   D. Stroke
   E. Tumor

3. The patient must be intubated, and maintained on intravenous midazolam to control seizure activity. What would not be an appropriate intervention in the ICU setting?
   A. Blood cultures, CBC, lumbar puncture, chest x-ray to identify a source of sepsis.
   B. Restore antiepileptic drug levels to therapeutic values
   C. Extubate the patient as soon as visible seizure activity ceases
   D. Urinalysis for myoglobin
   E. CT head with and without contrast

4. This is the patient's third trip to the emergency room in four weeks with seizure activity. Despite therapeutic levels of phenytoin, she continues to have frequent seizures. Phenytoin is the only medication she has used for seizures. Which of the following interventions would be least appropriate?
   A. Give more phenytoin until the patient complains of ataxia and tremor
   B. Add a second medication to her drug regimen
   C. Recommend a neurosurgery consult to resect the epileptic focus
   D. Recommend vagal nerve stimulator placement
   E. Tell the patient to stop taking her medication since it is not working

COMMENT

Initial treatment of status epilepticus • Status epilepticus is a neurologic emergency defined by 30 minutes of continuous seizure activity, or repeated convulsions without return to consciousness. Any type of seizure can persist as status epilepticus. The typical sequence of treatment begins by ensuring hemodynamic stability, followed by administration of a benzodiazepine to gain quick control of seizure activity. Thiamine, followed by glucose, and narcotic antagonists may be given with a suspected history of alcoholism or substance abuse, respectively. Fosphenytoin or phenytoin is given to establish continued control of seizures. If this fails, the patient can be intubated and given phenobarbital. With persistent seizures, the patient can be placed on a continuous IV drip of midazolam.

Causes of status epilepticus • The most common cause of status epilepticus, in a known seizure patient, is medication noncompliance. Other causes include alcohol withdrawal, traumatic brain injury, infection of the central nervous system, and cerebrovascular disease. Of course, status epilepticus may also occur without an identifiable cause.

ICU management of seizures and status epilepticus • Before extubation, the patient should show signs of return to normal consciousness after midazolam has been discontinued. Check the patient's EEG immediately to assure the patient has stopped seizing. Some patients with generalized tonic-clonic seizures continue to be in nonconvulsive status epilepticus without visible signs of seizure activity. The remaining listed answers are appropriate.

Treatment of refractory epilepsy • Helping a patient to gain control over seizures requires a work-up to determine the cause of the seizures, including a complete neurologic history and physical examination, brain imaging, and EEG. The dose of medication should be tailored for effective seizure control with minimal tolerable side effects.

Reasonable treatment options in this case would include increasing the dosage of phenytoin until either seizure-freedom or intolerable side effects occur. Another option would be to add a second anticonvulsant. Until a second medication is at therapeutic levels, the first medication should not be discontinued. The exception would be if the first medication is causing severe side effects (Stevens-Johnson syndrome, hypersensitivity reaction, or nephrolithiasis).

Once a patient has tried two or three anticonvulsants, evaluating the patient for surgical treatment would be appropriate. Surgical resection requires an identifiable seizure focus and a procedure that minimizes damage to important brain tissue. Alternately, the patient can be evaluated for a vagal nerve stimulator to reduce the need for medication.

Answers • 1-C 2-A 3-C 4-E

ACUTE RIGHT HEMIPARESIS

● CASE PRESENTATION

A 64-year-old female with a history of hypertension is brought to the emergency department by ambulance for evaluation of weakness of the right side and difficulty speaking. She had been well that morning and was found by her husband when he came home from work for lunch. He called EMS and she arrived in the ED 30 minutes later. On exam, she is hemodynamically stable with a blood pressure of 165/90. Fingerstick blood glucose was normal. Her general physical examination is unremarkable. On neurologic exam, she is alert and follows most simple commands. However, she has difficulty with word-finding and naming. There is weakness of the lower portion of the right side of her face and she has difficulty raising her right arm off of the stretcher. The strength in her right leg is relatively well maintained and left-sided strength is normal.

1. The most effective treatment for acute stroke is:
   A. Immediate anticoagulation with intravenous heparin
   B. Intravenous tissue plasminogen activator (tPA)
   C. Aspirin given orally or by suppository
   D. Lowering her blood pressure to less than 140/90

2. In considering the administration of thrombolytic therapy with tPA, the most important factor concerning her history is:
   A. Her age
   B. Her history of hypertension
   C. The exact time of onset of her symptoms
   D. The severity of her neurologic deficits

3. What is the most important single test to obtain quickly?
   A. Magnetic resonance imaging (MRI) of the brain
   B. Computed tomography (CT) of the brain
   C. Electrocardiogram
   D. Duplex ultrasound of the carotid arteries
   E. Complete blood count, coagulation profile, electrolytes

4. If she receives intravenous tPA, which of the following medications should be avoided for at least the next 24 hours?
   A. Aspirin
   B. Heparin
   C. Clopidogrel
   D. Antihypertensive medications
   E. A, B, and C
   F. All of the above

● COMMENT

Treatment of acute ischemic stroke • The most effective, proven treatment for acute ischemic stroke is the administration of intravenous tPA within three hours of the onset of symptoms to carefully selected patients. Strict criteria must be followed in selecting patients to minimize the risk of intracerebral hemorrhage (see guidelines issued by the American Stroke Association). Heparin has never been proven to have any efficacy in the treatment of acute stroke and does carry the risk of causing hemorrhage. Aspirin started within 48 hours of stroke onset has been shown to result in a small, but worthwhile improvement in outcome. Lowering blood pressure in the setting of acute stroke may frequently be deleterious because of a corresponding decrease in cerebral blood flow and is almost always the wrong thing to do unless other indications (such as concurrent myocardial infarction) exist for lowering it.

Contraindications to tPA treatment of acute stroke • TPA has only been shown to be safe and effective when administered within three hours of the onset of stroke symptoms. Thus, the exact time of onset of symptoms is critical in deciding about the administration of thrombolytic therapy. Elderly persons (>77 years old) and those with large neurologic deficits may be at increased risk for hemorrhage with intravenous tPA, but these are only relative contraindications and thrombolytic therapy may still be appropriate in some of these patients. While having a sustained blood pressure of greater than 180/110 is a contraindication, merely having a history of hypertension is not a reason to avoid the use of thrombolysis. Other important contraindications include a history of intracerebral hemorrhage, recent major surgery, and active bleeding or coagulopathy.

Testing needed prior to thrombolytic therapy for stroke • CT scanning of the brain to exclude intracranial hemorrhage is mandatory prior to the administration of tPA. It is also necessary to obtain the listed laboratory studies, but CT scanning and interpretation is usually the rate-limiting step in the management of acute stroke and thus high priority should be given to obtaining a CT as quickly as possible. An electrocardiogram or carotid duplex ultrasound is not necessary to decide about thrombolytic therapy.

Medications to be avoided after thrombolytic administration for stroke • Anticoagulants and antiplatelet agents should not be given in any form for 24 hours after the administration of tPA for ischemic stroke. Antihypertensive agents may be administered and blood pressure should be kept at less than 180/110 for at least 24 hours after tPA.

Answers • 1-B 2-C 3-B 4-E

CASE PRESENTATION

A 36-year-old auto mechanic presents one day after hurting his back on the job. While lifting, he experienced sudden pain in his lower back which tended to radiate into his left buttock. His co-workers took him to the emergency room where x-rays of his lumbosacral spine were unrevealing and he was sent home with instructions to take ibuprofen. He presents to your office the next day complaining of continued low back pain that also radiates down the posterior aspect of his left leg to about the mid-thigh. Physical examination is remarkable for some generalized pain and apparent muscle spasm in the lumbar paraspinal region bilaterally. Strength, sensation, and reflexes are normal throughout.

1. On the basis of his history and examination, you suspect the most likely diagnosis is:
   A. Lumbosacral strain (myofascial pain)
   B. Left S-1 radiculopathy
   C. Cauda equina syndrome
   D. Lateral femoral cutaneous neuropathy
   E. None of the above

2. The most appropriate diagnostic test to obtain within the next 24 hours in this case is:
   A. Nerve conduction studies and electromyography
   B. Myelography of the lumbosacral spine
   C. Magnetic resonance imaging of the lumbosacral spine
   D. Repeat x-rays of the lumbosacral spine with flexion and extension views
   E. None of the above

3. Which of the following physical findings would be most suspicious for a herniated disc leading to nerve root compression (radiculopathy)?
   A. Tenderness to palpation over the spine
   B. Tenderness to palpation and spasm of the paraspinal musculature on the affected side
   C. Loss of a deep tendon reflex
   D. Decreased vibratory sensation in the leg on the affected side
   E. None of the above

4. Appropriate management of this patient at this point would include:
   A. Reassurance, symptomatic treatment with a NSAID and/or muscle relaxants, and encouraging him to gradually resume his usual activities
   B. Advising strict bedrest for one week, then return for reassessment
   C. Referral to a pain specialist for epidural steroids
   D. Emergent referral to a neurosurgeon
   E. None of the above

COMMENT

Differential diagnosis of low back pain • Low back pain is one of the more common presenting complaints to physicians. Most acute pain syndromes are benign, self-limited conditions with the pain arising from myofascial sources. Patients with such conditions have a normal neurologic examination in spite of their pain complaints. Disc herniation, usually of the softer nucleus pulposus through the fibrous annulus of the disc, can result in nerve root compression. Clinically, this causes a radiculopathy typically manifested by radiating pain into the limb, sensory loss in the affected dermatome, weakness of the muscles supplied by the nerve root in question and diminished deep tendon reflexes in the territory of the affected root. Compression of the lower sacral roots and cauda equina can result in urinary and/or fecal incontinence. The lateral femoral cutaneous nerve arises from the lumbar plexus and supplies sensation to the lateral aspect of the thigh. Compression of this nerve as it crosses the anterior superior iliac crest can produce a condition of painful numbness affecting the lateral thigh known as meralgia paresthetica.

Evaluation of acute low back pain • Patients with back pain and normal neurologic examinations are unlikely to have any serious underlying pathology and further diagnostic testing is usually unrevealing. For patients with suspected radiculopathy, the best imaging study is likely to be MRI, although myelography followed by computed tomography (CT myelogram) can be useful (but more invasive). EMG/NCS studies can help if a peripheral nerve problem or radiculopathy is suspected. However, normal EMG/NCS studies do not exclude a radiculopathy. Plain x-rays of the LS spine are unlikely to be helpful in most cases.

Signs and symptoms of radiculopathy • Dysfunction of a specific nerve root (radiculopathy) may manifest clinically as pain radiating into the limb supplied by the affected root, sensory loss in the affected dermatome, weakness of the muscles supplied by the root (the muscles supplied by a particular root are known as a myotome), and diminished deep tendon reflexes in the territory of the affected root. Patients may exhibit some or all of these findings.

Treatment of low back pain • Most acute low back pain resolves within a few days without specific treatment. Symptomatic measures for pain relief may aid in shortening the course. Physical treatments such as physical therapy may also be symptomatically helpful. Studies have shown that prolonged bedrest is not beneficial. As long as the patient's neurologic examination remains normal, conservative therapy may be continued. Other, potentially more invasive strategies should be reserved for patients with neurologic dysfunction (especially weakness or incontinence) and with problems refractory to conservative measures.

Answers • 1-A 2-E 3-C 4-A

CASE PRESENTATION

A 20-year-old woman presents with a several months history of a coarse, proximal tremor involving both upper extremities. She also noticed progressively worsening slurred speech. Her family raises the additional concern of behavioral changes and notes that she seems quiet and withdrawn at present, in contrast to her usual open and outgoing personality. The family history reveals a maternal aunt who was diagnosed with liver dysfunction in her teens and later developed a gait disorder.

1. Based on this history and your thorough physical exam you suspect a hereditary disorder that can present with neurological, psychiatric, and hepatic dysfunction. Your working diagnosis is:
   A. Huntington's disease
   B. Pick's disease
   C. Wilson's disease
   D. Addison's disease

2. This disorder of copper metabolism is inherited in the following manner:
   A. Autosomal dominant
   B. Autosomal recessive
   C. X-linked recessive
   D. Sporadic

3. The following physical findings and/or test results support this diagnosis:
   A. Elevated free serum copper
   B. Low serum ceruloplasmin
   C. Low total serum copper and high urinary copper excretion
   D. Kayser-Fleischer ring
   E. All of the above

4. Possible treatment strategies include all except one:
   A. Zinc
   B. D-penicillamine
   C. Liver transplantation
   D. Manganese

COMMENT

Clinical features of Wilson's disease • Among the most common neurologic manifestations is tremor, which can have a "wing-beating" appearance when affecting the proximal upper extremities with more advanced disease. Other classic neurologic signs are dystonia, dysarthria, and gait abnormalities. Behavioral changes are common and many patients present with psychiatric features.

Pathophysiology of Wilson's disease • Wilson's disease is an autosomal recessive disease of copper metabolism. The affected gene on chromosome 13 codes for a copper transporting ATPase that is thought to be involved in hepatobiliary copper elimination and incorporation of copper into ceruloplasmin. Accumulation of toxic free copper leads to dysfunction of multiple organ systems.

Diagnostic testing in Wilson's disease • Testing reveals low serum ceruloplasmin and low total serum copper (reflection of reduced ceruloplasmin). Serum free copper is elevated, and urinary copper excretion increased. Virtually all individuals with CNS manifestations display a Kayser-Fleischer ring upon ophthalmologic examination reflecting copper deposition in Descemet's membrane.

Treatment of Wilson's disease • Treatment of patients with neurologic involvement initially requires D-penicillamine, a chelating agent that facilitates excretion of complexed copper into the urine. Maintenance treatment with zinc, which reduces copper absorption, may then be initiated. Orthotopic liver transplantation is a treatment option for patients with hepatic failure.

Answers • 1-C 2-B 3-E 4-D

CASE PRESENTATION

A 38-year-old man presents to the office with a chief complaint of nightly headaches, repeatedly occurring one to two hours after falling asleep. These began to occur about two weeks ago and he reports having similar headaches about the same time last year that resolved spontaneously in four to six weeks. While he has had an occasional headache during the day, these headaches more commonly awaken him from sleep, and last almost an hour. The headache is located behind the right eye, accompanied by tearing and nasal stuffiness. The intense pain causes him to become quite agitated until it resolves. Upon physical exam, his mental status, cranial nerve, motor, sensory, reflex, and gait exams are all normal. Touching the area over the right cheek, you are unable to elicit any painful response. There is no evidence of sinus disease, nor a history of neurologic deficits.

1. What diagnostic procedure would you like to perform?
   A. CT head, with and without contrast
   B. Lumbar puncture
   C. EEG
   D. EMG
   E. None of the above are indicated at this time.

2. What type of headache does this patient describe?
   A. Migraine with aura
   B. Tension headache
   C. Migraine without aura
   D. Cluster headache
   E. Trigeminal neuralgia

3. Which of the following medications would not be indicated for this patient?
   A. Sumatriptan
   B. Verapamil
   C. Oxygen inhalation
   D. Lithium
   E. Muscle relaxants

4. Which of the following triggers is commonly known to exacerbate these periodic headache cycles?
   A. Alcohol
   B. Exercise
   C. Foods rich in tyramine
   D. Application of ice
   E. Steroids

COMMENT

Diagnostic evaluation of headache • This type of head pain is classified among the benign headache disorders. No further diagnostic intervention is necessarily needed as the headache fits a typical pattern, and there is an absence of progression in severity, infection, neurologic deficits, or trauma. Any of the latter findings would necessitate neuroimaging, examination of CSF, and careful monitoring. The patient's complaints are not consistent with seizures, peripheral weakness or limb pain; therefore electroencephalography or electromyography are not indicated.

Differential diagnosis of cluster headache • The patient described here has the classic features of a cluster headache: unilateral, regular in periodicity, short duration, and accompanied by a partial Horner's syndrome that can include ptosis and miosis on the side of head pain. The typical profile of this patient is a 25- to 45-year-old male smoker, and the headaches are exacerbated by alcohol consumption. Behavior during a cluster headache reflects a desire to move around with the onset of head pain. This is in contrast to migraine patients who may experience a visual aura, unilateral head pain from 2 to 72 hours, and a desire to seek a dark, quiet room during the duration of the headache. Tension headache is a dull, persistent pain occurring in a bandlike distribution around the head. It is best improved by relaxation, stress management, avoiding triggers, or NSAIDs. Trigeminal neuralgia is described as lancinating pain provoked by mechanical stimulation in the distribution of the trigeminal nerve. Neuralgic pain responds to antiepileptic drugs such as carbamazepine (Tegretol).

Treatment of cluster headache • All of the medications listed in question 3 can be used, but muscle relaxants are the least effective. Oxygen inhalation at seven to eight liters per minute initiated at the beginning of the attack is considered one of the best therapies, as is subcutaneously administered sumatriptan. Verapamil and lithium are used prophylactically.

Headache triggers • Even in small doses, alcohol may precipitate cluster headaches as well as migraine. Cigarette smoking is also associated with cluster headache. Foods rich in tyramine may provoke migraine. Exercise and the topical application of ice are helpful for many different types of headache. Short courses of steroids may be used to treat refractory migraine or cluster headache. Women with migraine frequently note that it is worse at a particular time of their menstrual cycle.

Answers • 1-E 2-D 3-E 4-A

CASE PRESENTATION

A 71-year-old male presents to your office for follow-up after an emergency room visit for an apparent transient ischemic attack (TIA). He has a history of hypertension, glucose intolerance, and had experienced transient drooping of the left corner of his mouth and difficulty using his left hand, which resolved in about 5 to 10 minutes. By the time he was seen in the emergency room his symptoms had resolved and a CT scan of his head was normal. His medications include a diuretic for his hypertension and an aspirin a day, which he had started taking after he had some chest pain one year ago. His blood sugars seem to be controlled by watching his diet. He smokes less than one pack a day and has about one alcoholic drink a day. In the office, his general examination is remarkable for blood pressure of 152/93 and an irregular pulse, and his neurologic examination is normal.

1. The most important risk factor for stroke is:
    A. Cigarette smoking
    B. Alcohol consumption
    C. Adult-onset diabetes
    D. Hypertension
    E. Hyperlipidemia

2. Which of the following is not an appropriate first-line diagnostic test?
    A. Electrocardiogram
    B. Fasting lipid panel
    C. Carotid duplex ultrasound
    D. Magnetic resonance imaging
    E. Serum glucose level

3. Because of his irregular heartbeat on exam, you obtain an electrocardiogram, which reveals atrial fibrillation. The best approach to stroke prevention in this case would be:
    A. Continued treatment with aspirin
    B. Chronic anticoagulation with warfarin to a goal INR of 2.0 to 3.0
    C. Switch from aspirin to clopidogrel or extended-release dipyridamole/aspirin combination therapy because he experienced a TIA while taking aspirin
    D. Combination therapy with warfarin and low-dose aspirin
    E. Adding digoxin to his medication regimen and continuing aspirin

4. His carotid ultrasound reveals evidence of greater than 70% stenosis of his right internal carotid artery. The best approach to stroke prevention in this case would be:
    A. Chronic anticoagulation with warfarin
    B. Continued treatment with aspirin with the addition of an agent to lower his cholesterol and obtaining a follow-up carotid ultrasound in six months
    C. Referral for consideration of carotid endarterectomy
    D. Continued treatment with aspirin, adjusting his antihypertensive regimen to achieve better control of his blood pressure, and advising smoking cessation
    E. No change in his management is needed

COMMENT

Stroke risk factors • Nonmodifiable stroke risk factors include increasing age, male gender, positive family history of stroke, and certain racial groups such as African-Americans. Hypertension is by far the most important modifiable risk factor for stroke because it has a high prevalence and it increases the relative risk of stroke about fourfold. Other potentially modifiable risk factors for stroke include atrial fibrillation, carotid artery stenosis, cigarette smoking, diabetes mellitus, hyperlipidemia, heart disease, and physical inactivity. While heavy alcohol consumption is associated with an increased risk of intracerebral hemorrhage, light-to-moderate alcohol consumption has been associated with decreased risk of stroke compared to total abstinence from alcohol.

Diagnostic testing for TIA • While the diagnostic evaluation of a patient who has suffered a TIA has to be individually tailored to the case, the initial evaluation should be aimed at discovering modifiable sources of stroke risk and excluding conditions that require emergent or prompt treatment to avoid further problems. Thus, blood tests (CBC, coagulation parameters, electrolytes and glucose, cholesterol panel), electrocardiogram, and duplex ultrasound of the carotids are all indicated. The routine use of echocardiography to screen for a cardiac source of embolism is likely of limited use, although it may be extremely valuable in selected patients. While an MRI scan of the head provides more information, a CT scan is entirely satisfactory for initial evaluation of most patients with TIAs.

Stroke prevention in atrial fibrillation • Numerous clinical trials have demonstrated the effectiveness of chronic anticoagulation with warfarin to an INR of 2 to 3 in reducing the risk of stroke in appropriately selected patients with atrial fibrillation. Warfarin is clearly superior to aspirin, but aspirin is better than nothing for patients who are not good candidates for chronic anticoagulation.

Treatment of carotid stenosis • The North American Symptomatic Carotid Endarterectomy Trial (NASCET) has demonstrated the superiority of carotid endarterectomy over medical therapy alone for the prevention of stroke in patients with symptomatic (having had a stroke or TIA in the territory of the stenotic vessel) carotid artery stenosis of greater than 70%. The Asymptomatic Carotid Atherosclerosis Study (ACAS) found that carotid endarterectomy may be beneficial in reducing stroke risk in the setting of asymptomatic carotid stenosis, although this remains somewhat controversial. It is imperative that carotid surgery be performed by surgeons with low perioperative rates of stroke and death for the benefit of endarterectomy to be seen. It is also important to continue medical management of risk factors and antiplatelet therapy in patients who have surgery for carotid disease.

Answers • 1-D 2-D 3-B 4-C

CASE PRESENTATION

A 68-year-old retired physician presents complaining of memory loss. He casually describes occasionally forgetting to pay some of his bills and notes that he does have trouble remembering the names of new people that he meets. His wife is more concerned and notes that she has taken over paying the bills because his lapses are beginning to threaten their credit rating. She also describes an episode where a neighbor had to bring him home after he became lost walking the dog in their neighborhood. His past medical history is remarkable only for a history of moderately well controlled hypertension. On neurologic exam, he is alert and oriented except for some difficulty recalling the date. He is only able to recall one of three objects after a five-minute delay, but laughs this off and proceeds to explain to the examiner the intricacies of medical procedures he has performed in the past to demonstrate how good his memory remains. The remainder of his examination is unremarkable.

1. Cognitive decline in this age group is most likely secondary to:
   A. Normal aging
   B. Cerebrovascular disease
   C. Alzheimer's disease
   D. Depression

2. Appropriate diagnostic studies in this case would include which of the following?
   A. CT or MRI scan of the brain
   B. Neuropsychological testing
   C. Thyroid function testing
   D. Serum vitamin B_{12} level
   E. All of the above

3. Specific alleles of which of the following lipoproteins are associated with an increased likelihood of developing Alzheimer's disease?
   A. Apolipoprotein A
   B. Apolipoprotein E
   C. Lipoprotein (a)
   D. Low-density lipoprotein cholesterol

4. Which of the following classes of medications have demonstrated some effectiveness in treating the symptoms of Alzheimer's disease?
   A. Centrally acting cholinesterase inhibitors
   B. Dopamine agonists
   C. Anticholinergic agents
   D. Dopamine antagonists

COMMENT

Differential diagnosis of dementia • Alzheimer's disease is the commonest cause of dementia. Multi-infarct dementia secondary to cerebrovascular disease is the second leading cause of dementia. Other causes include thyroid disease, vitamin B_{12} deficiency, HIV infection, and neurosyphilis. In addition, depression in the elderly may manifest as apparent cognitive decline ("depressive pseudodementia") and should always be considered in the differential diagnosis of dementia. Healthy elderly generally exhibit little, if any, cognitive decline.

Diagnostic evaluation of the patient with dementia • The search for a treatable cause should be the primary focus of testing in a patient with dementia. Neuroimaging is useful to help exclude pathology such as chronic subdural hematomas or tumors affecting the frontal lobes that can cause personality change and cognitive difficulties. Laboratory screening for metabolic or infectious causes of dementia such as thyroid disease, B_{12} deficiency, untreated syphilis, and HIV as well as general metabolic and hematologic screening may be useful. Neuropsychological testing can help to characterize the cognitive deficits and aid in evaluation for underlying depression.

Genetic markers of Alzheimer's disease • While there is no specific diagnostic test for Alzheimer's disease, patients who carry the A4 allele of apolipoprotein E have been demonstrated to be at increased risk.

Treatment of Alzheimer's disease • Several different centrally acting acetylcholinesterase inhibitors have demonstrated modest efficacy in improving the functional level of patients with Alzheimer's disease. These medications seem to work best in patients with milder or early disease and are of less benefit in patients with more advanced Alzheimer's. Dopamine agonists and anticholinergic agents may be useful in the treatment of Parkinson's disease. Dopamine antagonists are useful antipsychotic agents.

Answers • 1-C 2-E 3-B 4-A

An Elderly Gentleman with Numbness in His Feet

● CASE PRESENTATION

A 68-year-old man presents to his primary care physician with a three-month history of progressive distal lower extremity weakness associated with numbness and tingling. There is a history of hypertension and some type of mild anemia but no history of diabetes mellitus or known toxic exposure. He notes some increasing gait unsteadiness over the past three weeks. Bowel and bladder function are preserved. Pertinent positive neurologic abnormalities include mild gait unsteadiness with positive Romberg. There is mild bilateral foot dorsiflexor weakness but intact power of the upper extremities. Deep tendon reflexes are slightly brisk in the legs with positive Babinski signs bilaterally. Sensory exam reveals questionably decreased pin and light touch to the mid-shin level bilaterally and with absent vibratory sense at the great toe and medial malleolus. Mild to moderately diminished proprioception is noted at the toes bilaterally. There is no spinal sensory level to pin when tested over the back region.

1. Differential diagnosis of bilateral lower extremity weakness in association with exaggerated deep tendon reflexes includes:
   A. Cervical stenosis, herniated cervical disc
   B. Amyotrophic lateral sclerosis (ALS)
   C. Subacute combined degeneration of the cord secondary to vitamin B_{12} (cyanocobalamin) deficiency
   D. Parasagittal meningioma
   E. All of the above

2. Diagnostic testing that may be of value includes:
   A. CBC
   B. Serum vitamin B_{12} determination
   C. HIV/RPR
   D. Cervical spine MRI
   E. All of the above

3. Low serum vitamin B_{12} levels have been associated with which of the following?
   A. Macrocytic anemia
   B. Peripheral neuropathy
   C. Subacute combined degeneration of the spinal cord
   D. Cognitive impairment.
   E. Isolated cerebellar atrophy
   F. All of the above, except isolated cerebellar atrophy
   G. All of the above

4. Treatment of vitamin B_{12} deficiency related to subacute combined degeneration of the spinal cord includes:
   A. Vitamin B_{12}
   B. Folate
   C. Ferrous sulfate, 325 mg by mouth twice a day
   D. All of the above

● COMMENT

Subacute combined degeneration of the spinal cord • Vitamin B_{12} deficiency may present with spinal cord disease. This syndrome has been referred to as subacute combined degeneration of the spinal cord and is manifested clinically as severe posterior column impairment and lateral cortical spinal tract dysfunction. Patients with spinal cord disease related to B_{12} deficiency have absent vibratory and position sense as well as hyperactive deep tendon reflexes with Babinski's signs. A positive Romberg sign as well as gait impairment are associated clinical findings. The differential diagnosis includes the cervical disc disease, amyotrophic lateral sclerosis, parasagittal meningioma as well as the other causes of myelopathy described below.

Evaluation of chronic myelopathy • The clinical picture described is consistent with a myelopathy. While chronic myelopathy can be secondary to B_{12} deficiency (often suggested by a macrocytic anemia), it can also be seen in structural lesions that affect the spinal cord which can be identified with MRI. Multiple sclerosis may present with a myelopathy and MRI may help with this diagnosis as well. Infectious causes of myelopathy include HIV, syphilis, and HTLV-I.

Effects of B_{12} deficiency • Neurologic problems associated with B_{12} deficiency include peripheral neuropathy, subacute combined degeneration of the spinal cord, and cognitive impairment or dementia. Patients may have neurologic manifestations of B_{12} deficiency even in the absence of anemia. Macrocytic anemia may occur before or after neurologic manifestations have become evident.

Treatment of the neurologic manifestations of B_{12} deficiency • Successful treatment and potential reversibility of the neurologic impairment depends on early diagnosis and prompt initiation of vitamin B_{12} therapy. This is usually provided as cobalamin, 1000 micrograms intramuscularly three times weekly for one month followed by lifetime 1000 micrograms intramuscularly once monthly.

Answers • 1-E 2-E 3-F 4-A

CASE PRESENTATION

A 56-year-old alcoholic male is brought to the emergency room by EMS after he was seen convulsing at a bus station. En route by EMS, his seizures were noted to involve his entire body, and were brought under control by IV benzodiazepines. He is lethargic, responds to pain, and incoherent. His serum blood alcohol level is only slightly detectable. He reportedly has no prior history of seizures. He has a normal neurologic exam with the exception of mental status changes.

1. Alcohol-related seizures are most likely to be:
   A. Generalized seizures, within six to 24 hours of the last drink
   B. Absence seizures, within three hours of the last drink
   C. Partial complex seizures, within three days of the last drink
   D. Status epilepticus, within two weeks of the last drink

2. The best management of alcohol-related seizures is:
   A. Phenytoin 300 mg at bedtime
   B. Treatment for alcohol withdrawal and abstinence
   C. Nothing because the seizures are self-limited
   D. Permitting occasional drinking, but not allowing binge drinking

3. Other metabolic causes of generalized seizures are:
   A. Hypocalcemia and hypercalcemia
   B. Hyponatremia and hypernatremia
   C. Benzodiazepine or barbiturate withdrawal
   D. Hypoglycemia
   E. All of the above

4. Of the following effects of alcohol on the brain, which is referred to as Wernicke-Korsakoff syndrome?
   A. Midline cerebellar atrophy with resultant truncal ataxia
   B. Nutritional deficiencies causing hypomagnesmia and hyponatremia
   C. Encephalopathy, ataxia, and nystagmus or ophthalmoplegia
   D. (C) plus anterograde memory problems
   E. White matter lesion in the pons associated with quadriparesis, gaze palsy, and mental status changes (central pontine myelinolysis)

COMMENT

Characteristics of alcohol related seizures • Alcohol withdrawal seizures are generalized seizures related to the acute reduction or cessation of alcohol intake in a person who is physically dependent on alcohol. If the patient demonstrates other types of seizures, they should be worked up for another cause of seizures (e.g., meningitis, stroke, trauma).

Treatment of alcohol related seizures • Since alcohol is a toxin, the best way to treat this type of seizures is to remove the offending source completely. Acute withdrawal treatment consists of sedation with a tapering course of benzodiazepines, thiamine, folate, and magnesium replacement, and rehydration. With extended seizure activity, the patient may be intravenously loaded with phenytoin, but this is tapered off after several days. Referral to a substance abuse treatment facility is appropriate.

Metabolic causes of seizures • Metabolic disarray is a frequent cause of seizures. Excessive or deficient sodium and/or calcium may be associated with seizures. Seizures may be caused by hypomagnesemia as well. Withdrawal from not only alcohol, but also benzodiazepines and barbiturates can result in seizures. Nonketotic hyperglycemia in addition to hypoglycemia may lead to seizures.

Neurologic complications of alcoholism • Wernicke-Korsakoff syndrome, described by answer D, is due to a thiamine deficiency (which also causes Wernicke's encephalopathy, described by answer C). Long-term alcohol use causes midline cerebellar degeneration. Rapid change in serum sodium can result in central pontine myelinolysis. Since many alcoholics present with hyponatremia, care should be taken to correct this slowly to avoid this potentially iatrogenic complication.

Answers • 1-A   2-B   3-E   4-D

CASE PRESENTATION

An 80-year-old, right-handed female is referred to your office for evaluation of headaches. She has a history of hypertension and osteoarthritis, but has otherwise been healthy. Her headaches began just over a week ago and are centered about the right side of her head. She has never really been bothered with headaches before and denies any recent lifestyle changes that could have triggered these headaches. She notes that the pain is relatively constant and waxes and wanes in severity. She has noted mild tenderness of the left side of her head when brushing her hair. She notes some increased pain when eating, especially down into her left jaw. When questioned, she also admits to some ongoing difficulties with pain in her shoulders and upper arms over the last few months. Her neurologic examination is unremarkable.

1. Other important historical points to ask about would be:
    A. The presence of fevers
    B. Any changes in vision
    C. Other focal neurologic problems such as weakness
    D. Any recent medication changes
    E. All of the above

2. Important points to check on physical exam include:
    A. Neck stiffness
    B. Palpable tenderness over the temporal arteries
    C. Visual acuity
    D. Examination of the oral cavity
    E. All of the above

3. Which of the following laboratory tests is most likely to be diagnostically suggestive?
    A. Serum glucose level
    B. Thyroid stimulating hormone levels
    C. Vitamin B_{12} level
    D. Urine drug screen
    E. Sedimentation rate

4. The most likely diagnosis is:
    A. Migraine headache
    B. Tension type headache
    C. Chronic subdural hematoma
    D. Temporal arteritis
    E. Fungal meningitis

5. This condition is best treated with:
    A. Triptan therapy
    B. Indomethacin
    C. Anticonvulsants
    D. Steroids
    E. Antifungal agents

COMMENT

Temporal arteritis (TA), historical points • Temporal arteritis, also known as giant cell arteritis, tends to be a condition affecting the elderly. TA is frequently associated with polymyalgia rheumatica, a condition resulting in chronic proximal upper extremity pain. This inflammatory process tends to affect primarily extracranial arteries, commonly branches of the external carotid artery. Patients may complain of claudicatory pain in the jaw while chewing. These patients are at risk of visual loss and more diffuse vasculitic involvement can lead to other serious complications.

Examination of the patient with headache • In addition to a complete neurologic examination looking for evidence of neurologic dysfunction, it is important to concentrate on several key features of the general examination of the headache patient. The head and neck examination is especially important. The scalp and skull should be examined looking for areas of deformity or tenderness. The ears and sinuses should likewise be carefully examined, especially for evidence of infection. Examination of the oral cavity may reveal evidence of a dental cause for the pain. The temporal arteries may become tender and inflamed in patients with temporal arteritis. The neck should also be examined for evidence of meningismus.

Confirmatory testing for temporal arteritis • The most useful screening test in patients with suspected temporal arteritis is a sedimentation rate. This is frequently, but not always, prominently elevated in TA. Confirmation of the diagnosis is obtained by temporal artery biopsy, which is usually performed bilaterally to increase the diagnostic yield.

Treatment of temporal arteritis • TA is treated with steroids. This treatment is necessary to help avoid severe complications such as blindness and stroke. Treatment may be initiated on the basis of an appropriate clinical history and elevated sedimentation rate and should not be deferred until pathological confirmation of the diagnosis. Temporal artery biopsy should be performed within one to two weeks of starting therapy with steroids.

Answers • 1-E 2-E 3-E 4-D 5-D

CASE PRESENTATION

A 42-year-old female with a history of renal transplantation four years earlier presents complaining of leg weakness and back pain. She had been well until the day before when she began to notice some pain in the mid-thoracic region and generally felt bad. That night, she accidentally urinated in bed while sleeping. The next morning she fell while walking to the bathroom and was brought to the emergency room for evaluation. On exam, her temperature is 99.9°F, and she is mildly tender to palpation over the thoracic spine. Her neurologic examination is remarkable for normal mental status, cranial nerves, and upper extremity strength and sensation. She is unable to lift her legs off of the stretcher and has diminished sensation from just above the umbilicus distally. Her reflexes are unobtainable in the legs and 1+ in the arms.

1. Findings suggestive of upper motor neuron dysfunction include:
   A. Increased tone in the extremities
   B. Hyperreflexia
   C. Extensor plantar responses (Babinski sign)
   D. Muscle fasciculations
   E. All of the above except muscle fasciculations
   F. All of the above
   G. None of the above

2. The best possible neurologic localization for her problem is:
   A. Myopathy
   B. Peripheral neuropathy
   C. Spinal nerve or nerve root
   D. Spinal cord
   E. Bilateral parasagittal cerebral cortex

3. The most likely diagnosis is:
   A. Guillain-Barré syndrome
   B. Polymyositis
   C. Herniated lumbar disc
   D. Transverse myelitis
   E. Spinal epidural abscess

4. The most useful diagnostic procedure would be:
   A. X-rays of the spine
   B. Nerve conduction studies and electromyography
   C. MRI of the spine
   D. Lumbar puncture
   E. MRI of the brain

COMMENT

Upper vs. lower motor neuron findings • Findings suggestive of upper motor neuron dysfunction include weakness, increased muscle tone, hyperreflexia, and extensor plantar responses. Findings suggestive of lower motor neuron dysfunction include weakness, muscular atrophy and fasciculations, and hyporeflexia.

Localization of a spinal cord problem • The best localization of this patient's problem is a spinal cord lesion in the mid-to-lower thoracic region. This is suggested by incontinence, a sensory level on the trunk, and bilateral lower extremity weakness. In the case of an acute spinal cord lesion, some of the usual upper motor neuron signs such as increased tone and hyperreflexia are not seen (as part of a syndrome referred to as "spinal shock").

Differential diagnosis of an acute, nontraumatic spinal cord lesion • The association of fever, back pain, tenderness to palpation, and neurologic findings consistent with a myelopathy is suggestive of a spinal epidural abscess, especially in this immunocompromised patient. While transverse myelitis could present in a similar fashion, the localized tenderness to palpation is more suggestive of an abscess. A herniated lumbar disc is more likely to produce signs and symptoms in the territory of a single nerve root. While Guillain-Barré syndrome and polymyositis can produce weakness, the presence of a sensory level on the trunk effectively eliminates these as diagnostic options.

Diagnosis of spinal cord problems • Currently, MRI is the preferred method of imaging most spinal cord pathology. It has the advantage of providing imaging detail of both bony and soft tissue structures. CT myelography may be helpful if MRI cannot be obtained emergently. EMG/NCS can help with the diagnosis of many lower motor neuron processes including radiculopathy, but cannot provide any specific information regarding spinal cord function. Abnormalities in the spinal fluid would not provide specific diagnostic information in this case where a structural abnormality affecting the spinal cord needs to be diagnosed or excluded. Lumbar puncture also has some potential risk for spreading the infection.

Answers • 1-E 2-D 3-E 4-C

HAND TREMOR IN AN ELDERLY MAN

CASE PRESENTATION

A 70-year-old man complains of worsening hand tremor. He has had a tremor since about 50 years of age, but finds it much more noticeable now. The patient reports that his father had a similar tremor. On neurologic examination a postural, symmetrical hand tremor that is absent at rest is found without any other abnormal neurologic signs.

1. Based on this history and examination your primary working diagnosis is:
    A. Parkinson's disease
    B. Rubral (midbrain) tremor
    C. Cerebellar tremor
    D. Essential tremor
    E. Orthostatic tremor

2. Which additional information about the patient's history would help support this diagnosis?
    A. Tremor ameliorated by alcohol consumption
    B. Tremor exacerbated by alcohol consumption
    C. Tremor awakens patient from sleep
    D. Tremor exacerbated by food consumption

3. Drugs that can cause or exacerbate tremor in this setting are:
    A. Lithium
    B. Dopamine agonists
    C. Beta agonists
    D. Neuroleptics
    E. Valproic acid
    F. All of the above

4. Medications with proven efficacy for this disorder are:
    A. Propranolol
    B. Diphenhydramine
    C. Benztropine
    D. Primidone
    E. Carbidopa/levodopa
    F. A and D
    G. All of the above

COMMENT

Differential diagnosis of essential tremor • Essential tremor (ET) is probably the most common movement disorder. Approximately half of the affected patients report a positive family history of ET. The tremor is characterized as a postural tremor, and is best seen with the affected body part in a fixed posture (although tremor also may be seen with action).

Characteristics of other tremor variants are: resting tremor in Parkinson's disease, goal-directed action tremor or intention tremor in cerebellar disease, mixed form (resting, postural, and kinetic) in rubral or midbrain tremor, and leg tremor upon standing in orthostatic tremor. In ET the hands are most frequently affected, followed by head, voice, and tongue. ET is thought to be central in origin with a possible tremor generator in the cerebellar-brainstem circuitry.

Effect of alcohol on essential tremor • ET is typically ameliorated by alcohol consumption. Patients may occasionally use small amounts of alcohol to help control their tremor in social situations such as dining out in public. Of course, tremor may be seen as part of the alcohol withdrawal syndrome. In this situation, alcohol may also lessen the tremor and this should not be confused with the therapeutic effect of alcohol on essential tremor.

Drugs that may cause or worsen tremor • Lithium, dopamine and beta-agonists, neuroleptics, and valproic acid are examples of drugs that can cause or exacerbate tremor in patients with and without essential tremor.

Treatment of essential tremor • Beta-blockers and primidone are pharmacologic treatments with proven efficacy for ET. Long-acting benzodiazepines may also be useful. Surgically implanted deep brain stimulators may be helpful for patients with severe unilateral tremor refractory to other attempts at treatment.

Answers • 1-D 2-A 3-F 4-F

CASE PRESENTATION

An 18-year-old college freshman is brought to the emergency room by paramedics after she was found unresponsive by her roommate. The roommate reports that the patient had complained of headache, body aches, and feeling like she had the flu last night. This morning her roommate found her lethargic and unable to get out of bed. Her temperature is 102 degrees, pulse 110, and BP 98/70. She responds to her name by moaning and only inconsistently follows simple commands. There is resistance to passive flexion of her neck. On pupillary exam, there is mild anisocoria with the left pupil about 1 mm larger than the right. Her face and all extremities move symmetrically and she withdraws from noxious stimulation with all extremities.

1. Which of the following diagnoses should be considered in this case?
   A. Meningitis
   B. Subarachnoid hemorrhage
   C. Drug intoxication
   D. Encephalitis
   E. All of the above

2. Following initial stabilization, which of the following procedures and/or tests are indicated emergently?
   A. CT scan of the head
   B. Lumbar puncture
   C. MRI scan of the head
   D. A and B
   E. C and B

3. A CT scan of the head without contrast is normal. Lumbar puncture shows 324 WBCs (primarily neutrophils), 12 RBCs, glucose of 23 (serum glucose = 78), and protein of 134. The most likely diagnosis is:
   A. Subarachnoid hemorrhage
   B. Viral meningitis
   C. Bacterial meningitis
   D. Fungal meningitis

4. The most appropriate initial treatment is:
   A. Neurosurgical consultation for aneurysm clipping
   B. Intravenous acyclovir
   C. Intravenous antibiotic therapy with a third generation cephalosporin and vancomycin
   D. Intravenous amphotericin B

COMMENT

Differential diagnosis of meningismus • This patient has altered mental status and evidence of meningeal irritation on exam. The two primary causes to be considered in this setting are subarachnoid hemorrhage and meningitis and they should be diagnostically ruled out before proceeding to other potential causes of altered mental status such as drug intoxication. Encephalitis is also a strong diagnostic possibility, frequently presenting with altered mental status, seizures, and fever (especially herpes simplex encephalitis), but would be less likely to present with associated meningismus.

Diagnostic evaluation of the patient with meningismus • Since subarachnoid hemorrhage and meningitis are the two primary diagnostic considerations, emergent testing should be directed at these two possibilities. CT scanning is very good for picking up evidence of acute bleeding into or around the brain and is quick and easy to obtain. MRI is more difficult to obtain emergently in most settings and acute intracranial bleeding may actually be more difficult to discern than on CT. If CT scanning is nondiagnostic and reveals no contraindication, then lumbar puncture (LP) should be performed looking for evidence of subarachnoid hemorrhage or infection. If bacterial meningitis is suspected, then antibiotic coverage should be started before CT and LP since these patients may rapidly worsen and culture results will not be altered on CSF obtained within a few hours of starting antibiotics.

CSF findings in meningitis • This spinal fluid formula is consistent with bacterial meningitis, showing elevation of the white cell count with a neutrophilic predominance, low glucose, and elevated protein. While the CSF in early viral meningitis can show an elevation in neutrophils (as opposed to a lymphocytic pleocytosis, which is typically seen later in the course of viral meningitis) and elevated protein levels, glucose levels are usually normal. Fungal meningitides could exhibit similar CSF findings, but the acute fulminating course in a previously healthy person is much more consistent with bacterial meningitis.

Treatment of bacterial meningitis • A third-generation cephalosporin plus vancomycin provides broad initial coverage for suspected bacterial meningitis while awaiting culture results and should be started emergently. Again, it is entirely appropriate to start antibiotic coverage before obtaining a CT or lumbar puncture, since patients with bacterial meningitis may deteriorate rapidly. Many would also start acyclovir in this setting to cover the possibility of herpes simplex encephalitis. However, this would not be appropriate therapy by itself since the CSF findings are more consistent with a bacterial process. Of course, antibiotic and antiviral therapy should ultimately be tailored to further CSF results. Viral meningitis generally requires only supportive treatment.

Answers • 1-E   2-D   3-C   4-C

CASE PRESENTATION

A 31-year-old female presents complaining of difficulty walking for the last two days. She had been well until two days ago when she noticed her legs felt somewhat "heavy" while going up a flight of stairs. Since then she has noticed progressive worsening of her gait. While she notes only a small amount of weakness, her legs feel stiff and she feels unbalanced when she walks. Her past medical history is unremarkable except for an episode of diminished vision in her right eye several years ago which resolved within a couple of weeks. Her exam is remarkable for an apparently sluggishly reactive right pupil compared to the left with otherwise normal cranial nerves. Motor exam is normal in the upper extremities and shows increased tone, but normal strength in the legs. Proprioception is perhaps slightly diminished at the toes bilaterally. She exhibits dysmetria in both the upper and lower extremities. Her reflexes are uniformly brisk with nonsustained clonus at the ankles bilaterally.

1. This patient's examination shows evidence involvement of which of the following parts of the nervous system?
   A. Right optic nerve
   B. Cerebellum
   C. Corticospinal tract
   D. Posterior columns
   E. All of the above

2. The history and examination is most consistent with which of the following?
   A. Guillain-Barré syndrome
   B. Multiple sclerosis
   C. Compressive myelopathy
   D. Cerebellar astrocytoma
   E. All of the above
   F. None of the above

3. Which of the following diagnostic tests is most likely to be helpful in this case?
   A. Nerve conduction testing and electromyography
   B. MRI of the brain
   C. MRI of the thoracic spinal cord
   D. Serum toxicology screen

4. This disorder is best treated with:
   A. Plasmapheresis
   B. Intravenous methylprednisolone
   C. Surgical decompression
   D. Radiation therapy

COMMENT

Neurologic examination in multiple sclerosis (MS) • In spite of improved diagnostic testing, MS remains primarily a clinical diagnosis that hinges on the concept of identifying lesions of the central nervous system that are separated in time and space. In this case, there is evidence of an apparent right optic neuropathy (probably the result of an apparent bout of optic neuritis several years ago), involvement of the posterior columns and corticospinal tract within the spinal cord, and abnormalities affecting the cerebellum and/or cerebellar tracts within the brainstem.

Differential diagnosis of MS • MS is an inflammatory disease that appears to have an autoimmune basis that affects the white matter of the central nervous system, resulting in focal areas of demyelination. While it can be chronically progressive, MS more frequently exhibits a relapsing-remitting course that may lead to accumulating disability. As noted above, the diagnosis rests on identifying lesions affecting the white matter of the CNS that are separated temporally and spatially as in this case. Guillain-Barré syndrome is an acute inflammatory polyradiculoneuritis that could cause gait difficulties, but which is associated with areflexia. A cerebellar astrocytoma or compressive myelopathy produce some, but not all of the symptoms in this case, and would not explain the prior history of monocular visual loss. Other conditions that may present similarly to MS include HTLV-I associated myelopathy, progressive multifocal leukoencephalopathy, neurosarcoidosis, inherited leukodystrophies, CNS vasculitis, and cerebrovascular problems such as multiple strokes or transient ischemic attacks.

Diagnostic testing in MS • Most patients with MS will have demonstrable abnormalities in the white matter of the brain, commonly in the periventricular regions and brainstem. MRI of the spinal cord is less commonly abnormal in patients with MS. Examination of the spinal fluid may also be helpful diagnosing MS with findings such as elevated IgG index and myelin basic protein as well as the detection of oligoclonal bands. Electromyography, nerve conduction studies and toxicology testing may help to exclude certain disease processes, but are not specifically helpful in establishing a diagnosis of MS.

Treatment of MS • Acute exacerbations of MS are best treated with steroids, which may shorten the duration of symptoms. Since an underlying infectious process such as a urinary tract infection may provoke worsening in MS patients, such processes should be excluded and/or treated prior to administering steroids. Several therapies are now available to help prevent exacerbations in patients with relapsing-remitting MS including interferon beta, glatiramer acetate, and mitoxantrone.

Answers • 1-E   2-B   3-B   4-B

CASE PRESENTATION

A 57-year-old man presents to his primary care physician with a six-month history of left upper extremity weakness predominantly involving the hand. He also notes reduced muscle bulk in both hands and a vague sense of weakness of the lower extremities. He has noted muscle twitching, cramping, and thinning of musculature of the right thigh. He has no sensory complaints. Cranial nerve examination is normal. Exam of the upper extremities reveals decreased muscle bulk of the intrinsic muscles of the left hand with thinning of the left brachial biceps. There is mild atrophy of the intrinsic muscles of the right hand. Fasciculations are seen over the shoulders and chest bilaterally. The right quadriceps muscle group appears of reduced bulk compared to the left. The left arm and right leg are moderately weak throughout. Reflexes are diffusely more brisk in the left arm than the right. Patellar reflexes are brisk and symmetric with downgoing toes bilaterally. Sensory examination is intact throughout.

1. Possible anatomic localization of the above neurologic abnormalities include:
   A. Cervical spinal cord
   B. Thoracic spinal cord
   C. Generalized peripheral nerve impairment
   D. None of the above

2. Diagnostic testing should include:
   A. EMG and nerve conduction studies
   B. MRI of the cervical spine
   C. MRI of the brain
   D. Acetylcholine receptor antibody determination
   E. A and B
   F. All of the above

3. The pathology of amyotrophic lateral sclerosis (ALS) includes involvement of:
   A. Spinal cord anterior horn cell
   B. Median motor and sensory nerve
   C. Spinal cord dorsal columns
   D. Lateral corticospinal tract
   E. A and B
   F. A and D

4. Which of the following are true of ALS?
   A. The cause of sporadic ALS is unknown
   B. The usual average duration of disease ranges from two to five years
   C. ALS is ultimately fatal, with death due to respiratory failure
   D. Patients with ALS can benefit from palliative care
   E. All of the above

COMMENT

Amyotrophic lateral sclerosis • This patient's neurologic abnormalities are most suggestive of a lesion affecting the cervical spinal cord. His presentation and examination are suggestive of amyotrophic lateral sclerosis (ALS) as a likely diagnosis. ALS has an average age of onset of 57 years with a male/female ratio of 1:7. The etiology is unknown. A common clinical presentation includes fasciculations and atrophy indicating lower motor neuron involvement, in combination with hyperactive reflexes, positive Babinski sign, and spasticity indicating upper motor neuron involvement. The unique combination of upper and lower motor neuron abnormalities is characteristic of ALS, but not specific for this enigmatic disorder. Sensory abnormalities are not seen in ALS. Structural spinal cord lesions can mimic this fatal condition and must be ruled out by careful attention to the neurologic examination and appropriate imaging studies.

Diagnostic testing in suspected ALS • Appropriate diagnostic testing also includes EMG and nerve conduction studies. MRI of the cervical spine is frequently an important test to rule out structural spinal cord disease. While this patient exhibited no cranial nerve abnormalities, MRI of the brain is useful to exclude structural brainstem pathology in patients presenting with bulbar involvement. The diagnosis of ALS is based primarily on clinical findings. It is therefore necessary to rule out potentially treatable underlying pathological conditions.

Pathophysiology of ALS • Pathologic anatomy includes severe loss of anterior horn cells, as well as degeneration of the lateral corticospinal tracts. The etiology of sporadic ALS is unknown. Current theories include oxidative stress resulting in death of spinal cord motor neuron cells (anterior horn cells). Familial ALS is less common than the sporadic variety and is associated with a mutation of the gene that codes for superoxide dismutase, type 1.

Treatment of ALS • Although cure is not possible at this time, it is important to provide psychosocial support for patients afflicted with ALS. There is a risk of patient abandonment and special care must be made to avoid this possibility. Risk of aspiration occurs when bulbar musculature is involved. Patients may elect to have a feeding gastrostomy. Palliative care support should be offered to patients with ALS. While specific curative therapy is not available, riluzole is a glutamate antagonist that has shown mild efficacy in prolonging survival of ALS patients.

Answers • 1-A 2-E 3-F 4-E

ACUTE COLLAPSE OF A MIDDLE-AGED MAN

● CASE PRESENTATION

A 56-year-old male with a history of poorly controlled hypertension is brought to the emergency department by paramedics after his family found him down at home. His blood pressure is 210/112 and his respirations are irregular. He is not responsive to questioning and does not follow commands. He has weakness of the left lower face and does not move his left arm or leg except to noxious stimulation. He exhibits semipurposeful movement of his right arm and leg. His CT scan is shown below.

1. The test most likely to demonstrate an underlying problem in a comatose patient with focal neurologic deficits is:
   A. Urine drug screen
   B. Serum electrolytes
   C. Lumbar puncture
   D. Computed tomography (CT) scan of the head

2. The CT scan shown demonstrates:
   A. An acute ischemic infarct
   B. Intracerebral hemorrhage
   C. An old ischemic infarct
   D. Subarachnoid hemorrhage

3. Intracerebral hemorrhage secondary to hypertension commonly occurs in which of the following locations?
   A. Basal ganglia
   B. Thalamus
   C. Pons
   D. All of the above
   E. None of the above

4. Which of the following measures may help to decrease intracranial pressure in this patient?
   A. Intubation and mechanical hyperventilation
   B. Intravenous mannitol
   C. Elevation of the head of the bed
   D. All of the above
   E. None of the above

● COMMENT

Evaluation of altered mental status • In patients with altered mental status and focal abnormalities on examination, imaging of the brain (CT or MRI) is usually the most helpful diagnostic test. In patients with altered mental status, fever, and meningismus, examination of the cerebrospinal fluid by lumbar puncture is usually diagnostically revealing when neuroimaging is not. Finally, patients with altered mental status and a nonfocal neurologic examination usually will have a metabolic or toxic cause for their condition.

CT appearance of intracerebral hemorrhage • Acute blood appears hyperdense on a CT scan. The image shows a hemorrhage in the right basal ganglia, not the subarachnoid space (Figure 3B). Thus, this is an intracerebral hemorrhage, not a subarachnoid hemorrhage. Infarcts initially result in mild hypodensity, loss of differentiation between gray and white matter surfaces, or may cause sulcal effacement. Acute infarcts may not be apparent on CT, but older infarcts typically become increasingly hypodense.

Location of hypertensive intracerebral hemorrhage • Hypertensive intracerebral hemorrhage typically occurs in regions of the brain supplied by small penetrating blood vessels such as the basal ganglia, thalamus, subcortical white matter, and pons.

Treatment of increased intracranial pressure • Hyperventilation, intravenous mannitol, and elevation of the head of the bed may all help to decrease intracranial pressure. The effectiveness of hyperventilation in reducing intracranial pressure diminishes within a few hours. While steroids may help to decrease vasogenic edema (such as that caused by tumors), they have no proven role in treating intracerebral hemorrhage or ischemic stroke. Patients with intracranial hemorrhage may also benefit from the ventricular drainage of cerebrospinal fluid to help control increased intracranial pressure.

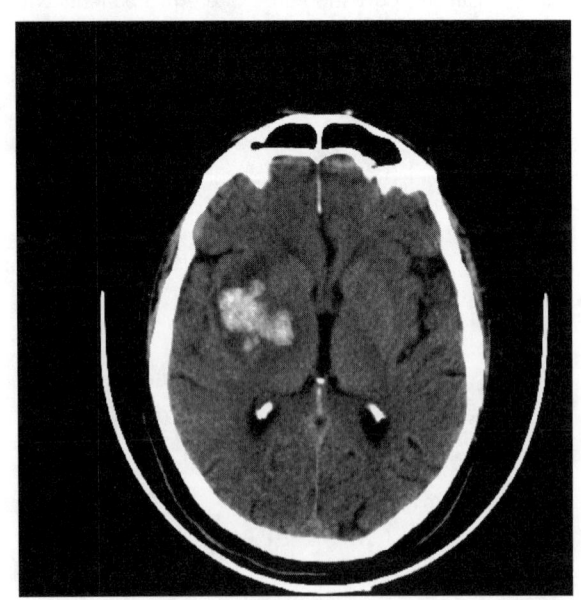

• Figure 3A

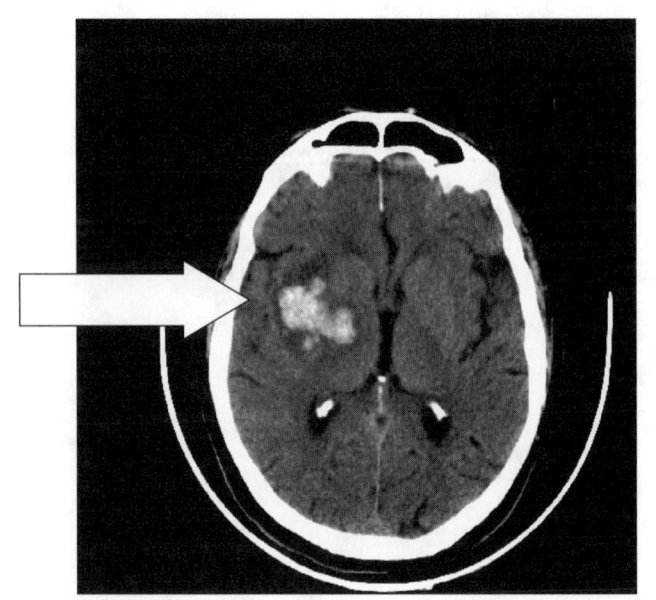

• Figure 3B

Answers • 1-D 2-B 3-D 4-D

Index

A

Acetaminophen overdose, 26
Acetazolamide, 10
N-Acetylcysteine, 26
Acute lymphoblastic leukemia (ALL), 11
Acyclovir, 24, 107
ADD. See Attention deficit disorder
Adenoidal hypertrophy, 25
Adenovirus, 44
Adjustment disorder
   hyperactivity and, 66
   sexual abuse and, 63
Adolescents. See also Children
   anorexia nervosa in, 30
   depression in, 36, 60
   epilepsy in, 95
   growth of, 49
   Guillain-Barré syndrome in, 7
   joint pain in, 56
   Osgood-Schlatter disease in, 48
   pneumonia in, 8
   pseudotumor cerebri in, 10
   puberty in, 35, 48–49
   SLE in, 56
   substance abuse in, 18
   vaginal bleeding in, 14
African-Americans
   cystic fibrosis and, 4
   depression and, 36
   stroke and, 100
Agoraphobia, 74
AIDS. See HIV disease
Albuterol, 31
   adverse effects of, 27
Alcohol abuse, 18. See also Substance abuse
   ADD and, 27
   cocaine and, 70
   irritability with, 80
   seizures and, 95, 103
   stroke and, 100
   tremor and, 106
ALL (acute lymphoblastic leukemia), 11
Allergies, 28
   drug, 95
   milk, 29
ALS (amyotrophic lateral sclerosis), 102, 109
Altered mental status, 107, 110
Alzheimer's disease, 83–84, 101. See also Dementia
   Down syndrome and, 39
Amblyopia, 51
Amenorrhea
   anorexia nervosa and, 30, 62
   primary, 47, 49
Amitriptyline, 82
Amoxicillin
   for otitis media, 9, 46
   for sinusitis, 17
   for UTIs, 23
Amphetamines, 60, 66, 93
Ampicillin, 23
Amyotrophic lateral sclerosis (ALS), 102, 109

Anemia
   alcohol-related, 80
   aplastic, 13
   hemolytic, 8, 53
   iron deficiency, 28, 41
   macrocytic, 102
   pernicious, 80
   sickle cell, 87
   toddler with, 29
Aneurysm
   berry, 93
   coronary artery, 46
Anorexia nervosa, 30, 47
   treatment of, 62
Anticholinergic toxicity, 82, 84
Antinuclear antibodies, 56
Anti-Smith antibodies, 56
Anxiety disorders
   hyperactivity and, 66
   hyperthyroidism vs., 79
   medical conditions and, 79
   phobia with, 73
   SSRIs and, 69
Aorta, coarctation of, 2
Apnea
   neonatal, 92
   sleep, 25, 28
Arrhythmias
   anorexia nervosa and, 30, 62
   stimulants and, 66
   subarachnoid hemorrhage and, 93
Arteritis, temporal, 104
Arthritis, 8
Asthma, 22, 31, 40
   classification of, 32
   flu shots and, 45
Astrocytoma, 108
Atelectasis, 40
Atherosclerosis, 100
Atrial fibrillation, 100
Attention deficit disorder (ADD), 18, 27, 61
   treatment of, 60, 66
Autism, 12
Avoidant personality, 73
Azathioprine
   for myasthenia gravis, 94
   for SLE, 56
Azithromycin
   for otitis media, 9
   for pneumonia, 8

B

Back pain, 72, 97
Bell clapper deformity, 20
Benzodiazepine, 95, 103, 106
Benzphetamine, 77
Benztropine, 90
Binging, 30, 62. See also Eating disorders
Bipolar disorder, 67
Blue dot sign, 20
Botulism, 91

Brain tumor
   dementia and, 101
   multiple sclerosis vs., 108
   seizures with, 88
BRAT diet, 44
Bulimia, 30
Bupropion, 69, 76
Burkholderia cepacia, 4
Burning pain, 82
Burr cells, 53
Buspirone, 69
Butterfly rash, 56, 81

C

Campylobacter spp., 44, 91
Carbamazepine
   adverse effects of, 82
   for seizures, 92
   for trigeminal neuralgia, 99
Carotid stenosis, 100
Catechol, 90
Cellulitis, 54
Cerebellar ataxia, 24
Cerebral palsy, 12
Cerebritis, lupus, 81
Cerebrospinal fluid (CSF), 93, 107, 110
Cerebrovascular accident (CVA). See Stroke
Cerivastatin, 86
Chicken pox. See Varicella
Children. See also Adolescents; Infants; Toddlers
   ADD in, 61
   adenoidal hypertrophy in, 25
   asthma in, 31
   depression in, 60, 64
   hemolytic-uremic syndrome in, 53
   Kawasaki disease in, 46
   leukemia in, 11
   muscular dystrophy in, 15
   nephrotic syndrome in, 54
   rhabdomyolysis in, 55
   scrotal pain in, 20
   seizures in, 6
   sexual abuse of, 63
   sinusitis in, 17
   Stevens-Johnson syndrome in, 5
   stroke in, 87
   thrombocytopenia in, 13
Chlamydial infections, 8, 49
Cholelithiasis, 4
Chorioamnionitis, 16
Circumcision, 23
Clarithromycin, 8
Clonidine, 76
Clopidogrel, 96
Clostridium spp., 44
Clozapine, 68, 90
Coagulopathy
   menorrhagia and, 14
   nephrotic syndrome and, 54
   stroke and, 87

Coarctation of aorta, 2
Cobalamin, 102
Cocaine abuse, 70, 93
Colitis
 HUS and, 53
 ulcerative, 47
Compliance, 68, 95
Conduct disorders, 63, 66
Condyloma acuminata, 567
Confusion, acute, 84
Congenital defects
 Down syndrome and, 39
 lithium and, 67
 pulmonary, 50
Congenital heart disease, 21, 39, 50
Constitutional growth delay, 33, 35
Corneal reflex, 51
Cor pulmonale, 25
Creatinine kinase, 55
Cremasteric reflex, 20
Crohn disease, 47
Croup, 3, 40, 57
Crush injury, 55
CSF (cerebrospinal fluid), 93
CVA (cerebrovascular accident). *See* Stroke
Cyclophosphamide, 56
Cyclosporine, 94
Cystic fibrosis, 4, 22
Cystourethrography, 23

D

Dehydration, 44, 52, 58
Dementia, 84, 90, 101–102. *See also* Alzheimer's disease
Dennie lines, 28
Denver Developmental Screening Test, 38
Depression, 18
 ADD and, 27
 adolescent with, 36, 60
 alcohol abuse and, 80
 child with, 60, 64
 criteria for, 37
 dementia and, 69
 eating disorder with, 30
 ethnicity and, 64
 sexual side effects with, 69
 SLE and, 81
Dermatomyositis, 56, 86
Desmopressin, 14
Developmental delays, 12, 38
Dexamethasone, 3
Diabetes mellitus
 burning pain with, 82
 Down syndrome and, 39
 gestational, 50
 obesity and, 77
 stroke and, 100
Diarrhea
 bloody, 53
 infant with, 52
 toddler with, 44
DIC (disseminated intravascular coagulation), 13
Diet, BRAT, 44
Diethylpropion, 77
DiGeorge syndrome, 21
Diphenhydramine, 82
Diphtheria, 45

Diplopia, 10, 94
Disc, herniated, 96
Disseminated intravascular coagulation (DIC), 13
Dog attacks, 74
Double bubble sign, 39
Double vision, 10, 94
Down syndrome, 39
 sleep apnea with, 25
 tetralogy of Fallot with, 21
Duke's disease, 58
Duodenal atresia, 39

E

Eating disorders
 anorexia nervosa, 30, 62
 bulimia, 30
Ebstein's anomaly, 67
Eczema, 28
Edrophonium test, 94
Electrolyte imbalances, 44
 anorexia nervosa and, 62
 rhabdomyolysis and, 55
Encephalitis, 107
Entamoeba spp., 44
Enuresis, 60
Epididymitis, 20
Epiglottitis, 3
Epilepsy, 6, 88, 92, 95. *See also* Seizures
Epinephrine, racemic, 3
EPS (extrapyramidal side effects), 68
Erythema multiforme, 5, 8
Erythema toxicum, 16
Erythromycin, 8
Escherichia coli
 diarrhea and, 44
 HUS and, 53
 UTIs and, 23, 84
Esotropia, 51
Essential tremor, 106
Exanthema subitum, 58
Exposure therapy, 65
Extrapyramidal side effects (EPS), 68

F

Failure to thrive (FTT), 4, 41
Fanconi syndrome, 13
Febrile seizures, 6, 58, 92. *See also* Seizures
Feet
 burning pain in, 82
 numbness in, 102
Fenfluramine, 77
Fifth disease, 58
Five *A*'s, 76
Fluphenazine, 68
Fluvoxamine, 60
Folate deficiency, 29, 80
Foreign body aspiration, 40, 57
Fosphenytoin, 95
Fractional excretion of sodium test, 52
Fruit juice, 41, 44
FTT (failure to thrive), 4

G

Gabapentin, 82
Gait disturbance, 15, 98, 102

Gastroenteritis, 44, 52
Gastroesophageal reflux, 22
Gastrostomy, 109
GBS (Guillain-Barré syndrome), 7, 91, 105, 108
Giant cell arteritis, 104
Giardia lamblia, 44
Glatiramer acetate, 108
Glomerulonephritis, 54
Glomerulosclerosis, 54
Glycogen storage diseases, 4
Gonorrhea, 49
Gower sign, 15
Growth
 adolescent, 33, 49
 charts of, 34, 42
 delay in, 33, 35
Growth hormone
 deficiency of, 35
 pseudotumor cerebri and, 10
Guillain-Barré syndrome (GBS), 7, 91, 105, 108

H

Haemophilus influenzae, 3–4
 immunization for, 45
 neonatal sepsis and, 16
 otitis media and, 9
 pneumonia and, 8, 40
 sinusitis and, 17
Hallucinations, 88, 90
Haloperidol, 68
Headaches
 alcohol abuse and, 80
 anxiety with, 79
 cluster, 99
 differential diagnosis for, 89
 hemiplegia with, 70
 migraine, 89, 99
 papilledema and, 10
 temporal arteritis and, 104
 tension, 89, 99
 triggers for, 99
Head circumference chart, 43
Heart anomalies, 2, 21, 67, 87
Heart disease
 congenital, 21, 39, 50
 obesity and, 77
 stroke and, 100
Heart murmur, 21
Helmet cells, 53
Hemangioma, respiratory, 57
Hemiparesis, 96
Hemiplegia, 70
Hemolytic-uremic syndrome (HUS), 53
Heparin, 96
Hepatitis
 antinuclear antibodies and, 56
 Guillain-Barré syndrome and, 91
 immunizations for, 45
 varicella and, 24
Hernia
 diaphragmatic, 50
 disc, 96
 incarcerated, 20
Heroin, 72. *See also* Substance abuse
Herpes simplex virus (HSV), 16, 107
Hip dysplasia, 39
Hirschberg reflex, 51

HIV disease
    dementia and, 101
    Guillain-Barré syndrome and, 91
    headaches and, 89
    myelopathy and, 102
    PCP and, 8
Holmes-Rahe scale, 78
Homocystinuria, 87
Horner's syndrome, 99
HSV (herpes simplex virus), 16, 107
Human herpes virus 6
    roseola and, 58
    seizures and, 6
Human immunodeficiency virus. See HIV disease
Human papillomavirus (HPV), 57
HUS (hemolytic-uremic syndrome), 53
Hyaline membrane disease. See Respiratory distress syndrome
Hydralazine, 56
Hydrocele, 20
Hyperactivity, 18, 27, 61
    treatment of, 60, 66
Hypercalcemia, 84
Hypocalcemia, 55
Hypochondriasis, 75
Hyponatremia, 52, 84, 93, 103
Hypospadias, 21

I

IBD (inflammatory bowel disease), 47
Idiopathic thrombocytopenic purpura (ITP), 13
Ileus, meconium, 4
Imipramine, 60, 66
Immunizations, 45. See also Vaccines
Immunoglobulin
    for Guillain-Barré syndrome, 7, 91
    for Kawasaki disease, 46
    for myasthenia gravis, 94
    for varicella, 24
Inborn errors of metabolism, 92
Infants. See also Neonates; Toddlers
    dehydration in, 52
    development of, 38
    dysmorphic features of, 39
    fever in, 58
    tachypnea in, 2
    tetralogy of Fallot in, 21
    tracheomalacia in, 22
    UTI in, 23
Inflammatory bowel disease (IBD), 47
Intracerebral hemorrhage, 96, 110–111
Intracranial hemorrhage, 96, 110–111
Intravenous pyelography (IVP), 23
Intussusception, 44, 58
Iron deficiency, 28, 41
Isotretinoin, 10
ITP (idiopathic thrombocytopenic purpura), 13

J

Joint pain, 56
Juice, fruit, 41, 44
Juvenile rheumatoid arthritis, 47, 56

K

Kawasaki disease, 46
Kayser-Fleischer ring, 98

Kidney stones, 95
Klebsiella spp., 23
Knee pain, 48

L

Lambert-Eaton syndrome, 94
Language delays, 12
Laryngeal papilloma, 57
Laryngotracheobronchitis, 3, 40, 57
Lead poisoning, 28
Learning disorders, 18, 27, 66. See also Attention deficit disorder
Leukemia, 39
Leukorrhea, 49
Levodopa, 90
Lewy body disease, 90
Liposuction, 77
Listeriosis, 16
Lithium
    adverse reactions to, 10, 106
    for bipolar disorder, 67
    for headaches, 99
Lumbosacral strain, 96
Lung function tests
    for asthma, 31–32
    for Guillain-Barré syndrome, 91
Lymphadenopathy, 11
Lymphoma, 47

M

Major depressive disorder, 37, 64. See also Depression
Malabsorption syndromes, 4
Malar rash, 56, 81
Malnutrition, 4
Maple syrup urine disease, 92
Marijuana use, 71
Mastoiditis, 9
Mazindol, 77
Measles, 45, 58
Meckel diverticulum, 29
Meconium ileus, 4
Membranous nephropathy, 54
Memory loss, 101
Meningioma, 102
Meningismus, 107, 110
Meningitis
    chemical, 93
    fever with, 58
    lumbar puncture for, 6
    treatment of, 107
Menstrual disorders, 14. See also specific types, e.g., Amenorrhea
Mental retardation, 12
Mental status, altered, 107, 110
Meralgia paresthetica, 97
Metabolism, inborn errors of, 92
Methadone, 72
Methylphenidate, 60, 66
Metoclopramide, 90
Midazolam, 95
Migraines, 89, 99. See also Headaches
Milk allergy, 29
Minimal change disease, 54
Minocycline, 10
Mirtazapine, 69
Mitochondrial disorders, 87

Mitoxantrone, 108
Moraxella catarrhalis, 3
    otitis media and, 9
    pneumonia and, 88
    sinusitis and, 17
Moro reflex, 38
Motor neuron dysfunction, 105
Movement disorders, 106
Moyamoya disease, 87
Multi-infarct dementia, 101
Multiple sclerosis (MS), 102, 108
Mumps, 45
Muscular dystrophy, 15, 86
Myasthenia gravis, 86, 94
Myasthenic syndrome, 94
Mycophenolate mofetil, 56
Mycoplasma pneumoniae, 8, 40
Myelomeningocele, 16
Myelopathy, 102, 105, 108
Myocardial infarction (MI)
    cocaine and, 70
    stroke with, 96
Myocarditis, 46
Myopathy, 86
Myositis, 86
Myringotomy, 9, 39
Myxedema, 35

N

Narcotics, 72, 83, 89. See also Substance abuse
Nasal polyps, 4, 17
Nefazodone, 69
Neonates. See also Infants
    respiratory distress in, 50
    seizures in, 92
    sepsis in, 16
    varicella in, 24
Nephrolithiasis, 95
Nephropathy, membranous, 54
Nephrotic syndrome, 54
Nerve conduction studies, 7
Neuroleptics, 68, 106
Neuropathy, peripheral, 82
Nicotine products, 76
Noncompliance, 68, 95
Nortriptyline, 76

O

Obesity, 77
Obsessive-compulsive disorder, 30, 60, 75
Olanzapine
    for bipolar disorder, 67
    for schizophrenia, 68
Olfactory hallucinations, 88
Omphalocele, 16
Opioids, 72, 83, 89
Oppositional defiant disorder, 66
Oral contraceptives, 14
Orchitis, 20
Orlistat, 77
Osgood-Schlatter disease, 48
Osteoporosis, 30
Otitis media, 9, 58
    adenoids and, 25
    Down syndrome and, 39
    Kawasaki disease and, 46
    pneumonia and, 8

P

Pain management, 83
Pancreatic enzyme replacement, 4
Panic attacks, 71, 79
Panic disorder, 74
Papilledema, 10, 58
Parachute response, 38
Parainfluenza virus, 3
Parathyroid hypoplasia, 21
Parkinsonism, 90
Parkinson's disease, 90, 106
Paroxetine, 65, 69
Patellofemoral syndrome, 48
Patent ductus arteriosus, 2
PCP. See *Pneumocystis carinii* pneumonia
Peak expiratory flow rate (PEFR), 31–32
Pemoline, 66
Peripheral neuropathy, 82, 86, 102
Peritonitis, 54
Personality disorder
    avoidant, 73
    obsessive-compulsive, 75
Pertussis, 45
Pharyngeal infections, 25
Phendimetrazine, 77
Phenobarbital, 92, 95
Phentermine, 77
Phenytoin
    adverse effects of, 82
    for alcohol withdrawal, 103
    for status epilepticus, 95
Pheochromocytoma, 79
Phobia, 74
    social, 73
Photosensitivity, 79
Pickwickian syndrome, 25
Pierre Robin syndrome, 25
Plaquenil, 56
Plasmapheresis, 91, 94
Pneumococcal heptavalent conjugate vaccine, 45
Pneumocystis carinii pneumonia (PCP), 8. See also HIV disease
Pneumonia
    atypical, 8
    delirium and, 84
    mycoplasmal, 8
    nephrotic syndrome and, 54
    recurrent, 4
    varicella and, 24
    wheezing with, 40
Poisoning
    acetaminophen, 26
    lead, 28
    vitamin A, 10
Polio immunization, 45
Poliomyelitis, 91
Polymyalgia rheumatica, 104
Polymyositis, 86, 105
Polyps, nasal, 4, 17
Porphyria, 79
Posttraumatic stress disorder (PTSD), 65
Prednisone, 94
Pregnancy, smoking and, 76
Primidone, 106
Progressive multifocal leukoencephalopathy, 108
Progressive supranuclear palsy, 90
Propanolol, 106
Proteus spp., 23
Proximal muscle weakness, 86
Pseudostrabismus, 51
Pseudothrombocytopenia, 13
Pseudotumor cerebri, 10
Psychosis
    parkinsonism and, 90
    steroid-induced, 81
Ptosis, 94, 99
PTSD (posttraumatic stress disorder), 65
Puberty, 49. See also Adolescents
    Osgood-Schlatter disease and, 48
    precocious, 35
Pulmonary function tests
    for asthma, 31–32
    for Guillain-Barré syndrome, 91
Purging, 30, 62. See also Eating disorders
Pyelonephritis, 23
Pyridostigmine, 94
Pyroxidine deficiency, 92

Q

Quetiapine, 68

R

Radiculopathy, 96
Rape, 65
RDS (respiratory distress syndrome), 50, 53
Reactive airway disease. See Asthma
Reflex(es)
    corneal, 51
    cremasteric, 20
    Hirschberg, 51
    Moro, 38
    primitive, 38
Renal failure
    anorexia nervosa and, 62
    dehydration and, 52
    rhabdomyolysis and, 55, 86
Respiratory distress syndrome (RDS), 50, 53
Respiratory hemangioma, 57
Respiratory syncytial virus, 3
Restless leg syndrome, 80
Reye syndrome, 26
Rhabdomyolysis, 55, 86
Rhinitis, allergic, 28
Rib notching, 2
Riluzole, 109
Risperidone, 68
Romberg sign, 102
Roseola, 58
Rotavirus, 44
Rubella, 45, 58

S

SAH (subarachnoid hemorrhage), 93, 107
Salmonellosis, 44
Sarcoidosis, 86, 108
Scarlatiniform rash, 58
Scarlet fever, 46, 58
Schizophrenia, 68
School failure, 18, 27
Scleroderma, 56
Scrotum
    pain in, 20
    swelling of, 54
Seizures, 88
    adolescent with, 95
    alcohol related and, 95, 103
    febrile, 6, 58, 92
    hemispherectomy for, 87
    hyponatremia and, 52
    neonatal, 92
    prolonged, 95
    stroke with, 88
    types of, 88
Selective serotonin reuptake inhibitors (SSRIs), 36, 60, 69
Selegiline, 90
Sepsis
    fever with, 58
    neonatal, 16
    nephrotic syndrome and, 54
Serotonin withdrawal syndrome, 69
Sertraline, 60, 65
Sexual abuse, 63
Sexual assault, 65
Sexual dysfunction, 69
Shigellosis
    diarrhea and, 44
    seizures and, 6
Shortness of breath, 71
Short stature, 33
Sibutramine, 77
Sickle cell disease, 87
Sildenafil, 69
Sinusitis, 4, 8, 17
Skeletal dysplasia, 35
Sleep apnea, 25, 28
SLE (systemic lupus erythematosus), 47, 56, 81
Smoking. See Tobacco use
Social phobia, 73
Spermatocele, 20
Spinal cord disease
    ALS and, 109
    degeneration of, 102
    localization of, 105
Spinal shock, 105
SSRIs (selective serotonin reuptake inhibitors), 36, 60, 69
Staphylococcal infections
    cystic fibrosis and, 4
    diarrhea from, 44
    pneumonia and, 40
Stature-for-age charts, 34, 42
Status epilepticus, 95
Steeple sign, 3
Steroids
    erythema multiforme and, 5
    for headaches, 99
    for multiple sclerosis, 108
    for nephrotic syndrome, 54
    pseudotumor cerebri and, 10
    psychosis and, 81
    for SLE, 56
    stress and, 78
    for temporal arteritis, 104
    for tracheomalacia, 22
Stevens-Johnson syndrome, 5, 8, 46, 95
Strabismus, 51
Streptococcal infections
    cystic fibrosis and, 4
    HUS and, 53
    neonatal sepsis and, 16
    otitis media and, 9

pharyngeal, 25
pneumonia and, 8, 40
RDS vs., 50
renal disease and, 54
sinusitis and, 17
Stress
　management of, 77–78
　posttraumatic, 65
　steroids and, 78
Stridor, 57
Stroke
　acute ischemic, 96
　child with, 87
　cocaine and, 70
　dementia and, 101
　migraines and, 89
　multiple sclerosis vs., 86
　muscle weakness after, 86
　risks for, 100
　seizures with, 88
　temporal arteritis and, 104
　TIAs and, 100, 108
　treatment of, 96
Subacute combined degeneration of spinal cord, 102
Subarachnoid hemorrhage (SAH), 93, 107
Subdural hematoma, 80, 101
Substance abuse, 18, 70. See also specific types, e.g., Alcohol abuse
　ADD and, 27
　back pain and, 72
　dependence vs., 18, 19
　irritability with, 80
　panic attacks with, 71
　seizures and, 95
　stimulants and, 66
　subarachnoid hemorrhage and, 93
Suicide, 26, 36, 60
Sumatriptan, 89, 99
Surfactant, 50
Sweat chloride test, 4
Syphilis, 101, 102
Systemic lupus erythematosus (SLE), 47, 56, 81

T

Tardive dyskinesia, 68
TAR (thrombocytopenia-absent radius) syndrome, 13
TCAs. See Tricyclic antidepressants
Temporal arteritis, 104
Tensilon test, 94
Testicular torsion, 20
Tetanus immunization, 45
Tetany, hypocalcemic, 55
Tetracyclines
　adverse reactions to, 23
　pneumonia and, 8
　pseudotumor cerebri and, 10

Tetralogy of Fallot, 2, 21
Thalassemia, 29
Thiamin deficiency, 103
Thrombocytopenia, 13–14, 53
Thrombocytopenia-absent radius (TAR) syndrome, 13
Thrombolytic therapy, 96
Thumb sign, 3
Thymoma, 94
Thyroid disorders, 4
　anxiety and, 79
　dementia and, 101
　depression and, 36
　diarrhea and, 44
　Down syndrome and, 39
　myopathy with, 86
　short stature with, 35
　tetralogy of Fallot with, 21
TIAs. See Transient ischemic attacks
Tick bites, 91
Tics, 27, 66
Tissue plasminogen activator (tPA), 96
Tobacco use
　ADD and, 27
　asthma and, 31
　bupropion and, 69
　headaches and, 99
　pregnancy and, 76
　stroke and, 100
Toddlers. See also Children
　acetaminophen overdose in, 26
　anemia in, 29
　croup in, 3
　cystic fibrosis in, 4
　developmental delay in, 12
　diarrhea in, 44
　failure to thrive in, 41
　otitis media in, 9
　strabismus in, 51
　stridor in, 57
Tonsillitis, 25
Tourette syndrome, 27
Toxic epidermal necrolysis, 5
Toxic shock syndrome, 46
tPA (tissue plasminogen activator), 96
Tracheoesophageal fistula, 22
Tracheomalacia, 22
Transient ischemic attacks (TIAs), 100, 108. See also Stroke
Transient tachypnea of newborns, 50
Transposition of great vessels, 2, 21
Tremor, 90, 98
　essential, 106
Tricyclic antidepressants (TCAs), 36, 60
　adverse effects of, 82
　migraines and, 89
　smoking cessation and, 76
Trigeminal neuralgia, 99
Trihexyphenidyl, 90

Trimethoprim-sulfamethoxazole, 5, 10
Trisomy 21. See Down syndrome
Truncus arteriosus, 21
Tumor lysis syndrome, 11
Turner syndrome, 2

U

Ulcerative colitis, 47
Urinary tract infections (UTIs), 23, 84, 108
Urine, maple syrup, 92

V

Vaccine(s)
　rotavirus, 44
　schedule of, 45
　varicella, 24, 45
Vaginal bleeding, 14
Vaginosis, 49
Valproic acid
　adverse effects of, 106
　for bipolar disorder, 67
　for migraines, 89
Vampires, 79
Vancomycin, 107
Varicella, 24, 45, 87
Varicocele, 20
Venlafaxine, 60, 69
Ventriculoperitoneal shunting, 10
Verapamil, 99
Vitamin A toxicity, 10
Vitamin B_{12} deficiency, 80, 101, 102
Voiding cystourethrography (VCUG), 23
Von Willebrand disease, 14

W

Warfarin, 100
Weight-for-age charts, 34, 42
Weight-for-length chart, 43
Wernicke-Korsakoff syndrome, 103
Wheezing, 22, 40
Wilson's disease, 98

Y

Yersinia enterocolitica, 47

Z

Zinc, 98
Ziprasidone, 68
Zoster. See Varicella
Zyban, 76